PRAISE FOR
DECODE YOUR FATIGUE

'A hopeful, practical book to help people move from
debilitating fatigue to a purposeful, joyful life once again.'

MIRANDA HART, COMEDIAN, ACTOR, AND WRITER

'Are you ready to be empowered instead of blown off? Enlightened,
instead of fumbling in the dark? Here is a map to help you get
there. From somebody healthy, who has been where you are!'

JACOB TEITELBAUM, M.D., AUTHOR OF THE BEST-SELLING *FROM FATIGUED TO FANTASTIC!*

'Alex Howard, and his colleagues, have been doing exceptional
work with patients and clients with various types of persistent
fatigue for many years. Fatigue is an immensely complex issue
to investigate and properly address clinically, and this book does
a masterful job of tackling these complexities and discussing
them in a format and style that it easily understood and relatable
for the layperson and medical professional alike. Bravo!'

PROFESSOR DR. DAVID BRADY, AUTHOR OF *THE FIBRO-FIX*

'In writing this book Alex shows how Western medicine is failing
patients with CFS/ME. Doctors do not look for disease causation nor
try to identify the mechanisms by which that person has become ill.
In Decode Your Fatigue, Alex gives the reader a roadmap and explains
how symptoms can be used as important direction finders to guide
recovery. With the rules of recovery and the tools to fix, all is possible.
The tools are within everyone's grasp and the book is logical so difficult
concepts are easily understood. Yes, this is not an easy journey, it takes
determination and courage. But with Decode Your Fatigue you can do it.'

DR. SARAH MYHILL, AUTHOR OF *DIAGNOSIS AND TREATMENT OF CHRONIC FATIGUE
SYNDROME AND MYALGIC ENCEPHALITIS: IT'S MITOCHONDRIA, NOT HYPOCHONDRIA*

T0286329

"Finally, a practical guide to recovery from fatigue that is not only inspiring but also very doable. Each of the different systems that are involved in fatigue are covered. Decode Your Fatigue teaches you how to personalize your healing journey, which is so very important because each of us is quite unique. Thank you, Alex, for this comprehensive roadmap to recovery! Highly recommended!"

DONNA GATES, M. ED., ABAAHP,
INTERNATIONAL BESTSELLING AUTHOR OF THE BODY ECOLOGY DIET

'I am deeply appreciative of Alex and his team's work at OHC. There are a lot of books about fatigue. So many that you may want to skip this one – but I implore you: DON'T! Let this be the book you pick up and read. Alex's approach to deep, lasting, multifactorial, complex fatigue is different. Yes, it started with his own experience, but it evolved to him establishing a clinic with a committed research department and a team of brilliant, like-minded individuals all drilling down into different aspects of the fatigue puzzle. Not only have they treated thousands of patients successfully over the decades, but they've published many research studies on their approach. Regardless of the underlying cause of your fatigue, if you give this book the time – and your precious energy – it will likely be the last stop you'll need to make on the long, often deeply discouraging journey of healing from chronic fatigue.'

DR KARA FITZGERALD, CLINIC DIRECTOR AND HOST OF THE 'NEW
FRONTIERS IN FUNCTIONAL MEDICINE' PODCAST

'Decode Your Fatigue provides an extraordinary opportunity for the reader to finally feel understood, validating what we might be experiencing with our health challenges and symptoms related to the lack of energy. Alex provides an easy 12-step process that cultivates hope for achieving recovery. This is a must read for anyone suffering from chronic fatigue or other similar ailments, and will become a staple in our clinic and in our practitioner education'

ANDREA NAKAYAMA, MSN, FNLP, CNE, CNC, FUNCTIONAL MEDICINE NUTRITIONIST,
FOUNDER AND CLINICAL DIRECTOR, FUNCTIONAL NUTRITION ALLIANCE

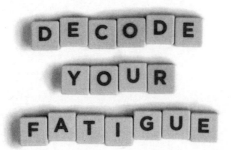

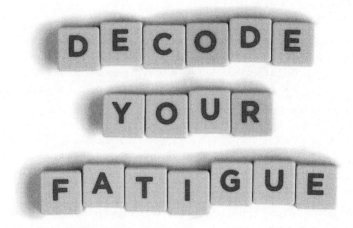

A Clinically Proven 12-Step Plan
to Increase Your Energy, Heal Your Body,
and Transform Your Life

Alex Howard

HAY HOUSE

Carlsbad, California • New York City
London • Sydney • New Delhi

Published in the United Kingdom by:
Hay House UK Ltd, The Sixth Floor, Watson House,
54 Baker Street, London W1U 7BU
Tel: +44 (0)20 3927 7290; Fax: +44 (0)20 3927 7291; www.hayhouse.co.uk

Published in the United States of America by:
Hay House Inc., PO Box 5100, Carlsbad, CA 92018-5100
Tel: (1) 760 431 7695 or (800) 654 5126
Fax: (1) 760 431 6948 or (800) 650 5115; www.hayhouse.com

Published in Australia by:
Hay House Australia Pty Ltd, 18/36 Ralph St, Alexandria NSW 2015
Tel: (61) 2 9669 4299; Fax: (61) 2 9669 4144; www.hayhouse.com.au

Published in India by:
Hay House Publishers India, Muskaan Complex,
Plot No.3, B-2, Vasant Kunj, New Delhi 110 070
Tel: (91) 11 4176 1620; Fax: (91) 11 4176 1630; www.hayhouse.co.in

Tradepaper ISBN: 978-1-4019-6110-7
E-book ISBN: 978-1-78817-461-9
Audiobook ISBN: 978-1-78817-603-3

10 9 8 7 6 5 4 3 2 1

Interior illustrations: iii, v, 1, 59, 139: Antigone Konstantinidou; all other images:
Sam Smith

Printed in the United States of America

▪▪ CONTENTS ▪▪

PART III: RECOVERING FROM FATIGUE

Part I

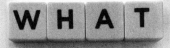

WHAT

IS

FATIGUE?

Chapter 1

RADICAL RESPONSIBILITY

L ike most people, I grew up believing that if you fall ill, you take a pill and you feel better. At least that was until just before my 16th birthday, when I found myself in a physical hell that no pill could cure.

I woke up one morning and something felt very wrong. It was as though someone had pulled the plug on the energy in my body, and I had none left. The short walk from my bedroom to the bathroom felt like a marathon, my muscles ached, and I became light-headed while doing even the most basic tasks.

Following several visits to the doctor and various blood tests, it was concluded that I had a virus. I just needed to rest, I was told, and all would be back to normal in a month or two. That felt like a lifetime for a teenage boy who just wanted to play sports and make music with his friends.

For a while ignorance wasn't exactly bliss, but it never crossed my mind that what I was experiencing was anything more sinister than a virus that would pass in its own time. Except, it didn't...

Three months later, I was heading to the doctor once more in search of answers. This time, my grandmother was leading the charge – if anyone could get answers, it was her. My health hadn't improved since my last appointment; in fact, it'd declined significantly. An attempt to restart school a few weeks earlier had gone horribly wrong: after 10 days of pushing through and pretending there was nothing wrong with me, I'd crashed, and was now feeling worse than ever.

The doctor's surgery (office) was only a five-minute drive from our home but it might as well have been a million miles away. By the time we arrived I was so dizzy I could hardly stand and the exhaustion was so crippling it took everything I had not to just lie on the floor and curl up in a ball.

As we sat in the waiting room, I tried to distract myself by scanning the other patients. With a strange kind of envy, I found myself wishing I could swap my illness for a more tangible condition. I'd willingly have taken a broken limb or some kind of unpleasant infectious disease because they at least have a clear recovery path. The lack of clarity on my own way forward was almost as bad as my crippling symptoms.

When I was called in to see the doctor, my grandmother accompanied me. As I completed my description of the latest developments, or lack thereof, she interrupted: 'Do you think it could be chronic fatigue syndrome, or ME?' she asked the doctor, in the slightly overassertive voice someone uses when they realize they might be speaking out of turn.

A long pause followed, during which the doctor's face assumed a somewhat pensive expression. My slower than normal brain used this interval to try and make sense of what my grandmother had just suggested. I didn't know much about chronic fatigue syndrome, but I understood it was bad news and that it was a diagnosis I didn't want.

Eventually, the doctor responded: 'Yes, I think that's the most likely explanation.'

After another pause, I stepped in. 'Well, what does that mean?' I asked. 'Is there a pill I can take or something?'

'No, I'm afraid there is nothing I can give you,' he replied. 'The best I can offer is counseling.'

As I struggled to process the enormity of what the doctor was telling me – that I had a serious condition for which nothing could be done – his suggestion that I have counseling stung deeply. I wanted to shout and scream about how ridiculous it was, but I didn't have the energy. How could he be so insulting? My illness was in my body, not my mind.

The Downside of Hope

It would take several years before the horror of that autumn morning fully sank in. As the months passed, my grandmother, unwilling to accept that conventional medicine couldn't provide a solution to my condition, dragged me around the weird and wonderful local alternative healthcare scene: nutritionists, energy healers, Chinese and Indian medicine practitioners... I saw them all.

I remember feeling genuinely hopeful and excited on the first few occasions; however, a clear and predictable pattern soon emerged. The virtues of the latest offering would be described to me, and I'd read a leaflet that included testimonials from people with symptoms like my own. I'd suspend my disbelief and become optimistic that the treatment would work, only to be disappointed once more when a few weeks or months later it became clear that it wasn't making a blind bit of difference.

In time, I stopped getting my hopes up. Not because I didn't want to get better – I did, I wanted it more than anything – but because I could no longer handle the emotional roller coaster of disappointment. I wasn't cynical by nature but I became cynical because it was the only way I could protect myself from the downside of hope.

Over the next two years I saw numerous supposed medical experts; I radically transformed my diet; I had more blood tests than I was aware existed; and I consulted everyone from faith healers to people I'm not sure were medically sane – all to no avail. If anything, my symptoms got worse, and after a prolonged period in this living hell, my mindset certainly did.

The Turning Point

My health reached its lowest ebb when I was 18. And while it wouldn't be true to say I was suicidal – because I didn't want to die – at the same time, I just couldn't see a way to keep living in the nightmare my life had become. I was in pain every day, and sometimes taking the few steps from my bedroom to the bathroom felt like climbing Mount Everest. It was in this state of desperation that I picked up the phone one day and called my uncle, and had the conversation that would change the course of my life.

My uncle was a bit like Gandalf in *Lord of the Rings* – he wasn't around very often but he did have a sneaky habit of turning up at just the right time with just the right words of advice, before disappearing again over the horizon. I'd learnt to deeply admire and respect him from a distance, and the fact that he ran an indie record label also made him very cool to an aspiring punk-rock guitarist like myself.

When you have a severe chronic illness it's not so easy to rely on the usual pleasantries when beginning a conversation. The seemingly innocuous question 'How are you?' has multifaceted answers and 'I'm fine, thank you,' as polite and normal as it sounds, is a blatant lie. 'Fine' falls into the same category as 'pleasant' or 'amiable.' It can refer more to the absence of something than to its presence.

However, by that stage in my illness I was past the point of caring what other people thought of me. Without the energy left to hold back, I told my uncle exactly how I felt: I hated my life and everything in it; I didn't want to face another day of the hell my life had become; I was at the end of my tether and I couldn't take much more.

Now, one would typically expect a response of compassion and gentleness in such a situation, and it wasn't that my uncle didn't know that I deserved both – he did. But he also realized that tea-and-biscuits sympathy wasn't going to change anything. He knew that, as hard as it might seem, if I wanted the circumstances of my life to change, I was going to have to change them *myself*.

He started off by asking me a simple question: 'On a scale of 0 to 10, how badly do you want to get better'? I didn't have to think about it for long. I believed I'd do virtually anything – short of murder or amputating one of my limbs – to get better. I decided I was a 9½ out of 10. My next task was to make a list of all the things I thought I could *do* to get better, followed by a list of all the things that made me worse. My uncle suggested I put down the phone and come up with these two lists before calling him back in 10 minutes.

As I compiled my list of the things I could do to get better, I uncovered all kinds of excuses: I'd already tried everything and nothing had worked, and how was I supposed to find answers when no one else had? However, I respected my uncle and I was also desperate, so I listed things like meditation and yoga and learning more about food and nutrition; I even wrote 'exploring more about psychology' – I was *that* desperate.

I then worked on my list of things that made me worse. I had just one word: life. It felt as if trying to get through the day was its own unique source of torture.

I called my uncle, feeling proud that I'd at least bothered to do the exercise. I walked him through my lists, and he pointed out that part of what I needed to do was dig deeper to find answers. However, it was his next two questions that changed everything for me. 'How many hours a day do you spend doing the things that you believe could make a difference?' he asked.

My answer was as pathetic as it sounded. It was, basically, *none*. I knew of things I could be doing – they were on my list, after all – but the truth was, I wasn't doing them.

He then asked, without a hint of judgment: 'How many hours a day do you spend watching television?' I took a moment to calculate the number of soap operas I sat through, along with various other mindless TV shows, and rather sheepishly, gave him my answer: I was watching TV for around seven hours a day. I had my excuses of course: I didn't have the energy to do anything else and it helped numb my mind while my body was so ill.

My uncle then revealed the carefully poised point he wanted to make: 'So, you want to get better on a scale of 9½ out of 10, and you'd do almost anything to achieve it. You have a list of things that could possibly help you, although you don't spend any time doing them. However, you do have seven hours a day that you spend watching television.'

'Something doesn't quite add up there, does it?' he concluded, with just enough softness and heart that, rather than becoming defensive, I found myself thinking long and hard.

Over the next hour, my uncle helped me draw up a plan that would change everything for me. From that moment on, with a depth of determination that surprises me to this day, I committed myself to finding a path to recovery. I gave it *everything*. My healing journey consumed my entire life; I was so desperate, I felt I had no other choice.

Decoding My Fatigue

Over the next five years, I saw more than 30 different practitioners, I read more than 500 books, and I practiced meditation and yoga for thousands of hours. Along the way it struck me that recovering from fatigue is like decoding a cryptic puzzle – you need to apply the right interventions, in the right sequence, at the right time.

My recovery path involved seemingly endless trial and error, and at times trying to make sense of things was beyond frustrating. In time, it became clear to me that putting things together in the right way can be as important as having the right ingredients: I found that treatments that are helpful at one stage of recovery can make things worse at another stage. Long before the concept of biohacking gained currency in popular culture, in a sense that was what I was doing – running endless experiments on my body to slowly decode the puzzle of my fatigue.

Five years after that fateful conversation with my uncle, I finally knew that I'd fully recovered. I believe that everyone who goes through an experience like mine has a measure for this, where they think, *If I could do that without payback, then I'd know I'm fully recovered.*

For me, *that* was going for a full-on run and holding nothing back. If you'd seen me that day, I'm sure you'd have agreed it really wasn't far off that iconic scene in *Rocky*. I ascended one of the steepest hills in London, giving it my all, and I was in tears by the time I reached the top. However, the run itself wasn't the real test of my recovery – that came in the days that followed when, instead of the physical payback that's so typical of chronic fatigue, I felt nothing but ready to go again.

Founding The Optimum Health Clinic

In the later years of my recovery, I studied for a degree in psychology in Wales, and as part of my final-year research, I interviewed 10 people who, like me, had personal experience of severe fatigue, to understand how it'd impacted their sense of self. The three who'd recovered reported that in spite of the immense difficulty and suffering they'd endured, their lives had been enriched by the experience. This is something that's referred to academically as post-traumatic growth.[1]

And although I'd have found it very hard to accept it when I was at my most desperate, I knew the same was true for me. Having been to hell and back, I'd learned things about myself and the world that gave me a powerful sense of my own capacity, along with a deep sense of my responsibility to help people in a similar situation.

So, after a year of working as an apprentice to one of my psychology trainers, I decided to set up the kind of clinic that I'd wished had existed in the years I'd been ill. Fueled by little more than a passion to help and the belief that I'd found some of the answers along the way, I launched The Optimum Health Clinic (OHC) from my bedsit in North London, at a time when making the rent each month was a serious struggle.

Within a few months, I'd received *thousands* of inquiries from people all over the UK who were suffering from myalgic encephalomyelitis (ME), chronic fatigue syndrome (CFS), and fibromyalgia. In time, I invited a nutritional therapist, Niki Gratrix, to join me – although I had a good basic knowledge of nutrition, I knew that my specialty was psychology.

And, as things grew beyond what Niki and I could handle on our own, we were joined by Anna Duschinsky, who became our Director of Psychology, allowing me to focus on the overall vision and leadership of the clinic. Anna had a very similar healing story to my own, and our personal experiences became a critical part of our patient-centered approach.

It was an immensely exciting time, but it came with a great burden of responsibility. From day one, we were determined not to fall into the trap of claiming that we had all the answers, or that ours was the only approach to fatigue that mattered, as many other practitioners had done. With a maturity that was in many ways beyond our years, we carefully crafted a game-changing approach to treating fatigue-related conditions that places the individual differences of each patient at the heart of everything.

In the early years of the OHC, finding, training, and supporting the best practitioner team possible presented so many challenges. Aside from an A level in business studies, I had no experience of business, and indeed, had never even held a 'proper' job. We were continually learning as we worked, and looking back now I think it's something of a miracle that we managed to survive the rocket-ship growth we experienced at times.

Thankfully, we seemed to attract the right people at just the right time to help guide and support us, a blessing that has sustained us to this very day. And, as it happens, you'll meet some of them while reading this book.

In time it became super clear to us that if we wanted our approach to fatigue-related conditions to ultimately be accepted by and integrated into mainstream medicine, we needed to talk the language of medicine, otherwise known as the language of research. And so in 2011 we founded our own research department.

A year later we published a prospective preliminary study in the *British Medical Journal Open* that demonstrated statistically significant improvement with our approach.[2] We followed this up with publications in *Psychology and Health, Medical Hypotheses,* and the *Journal of Integral Theory and Practice,* to name but a few.[3]

In the years since, the OHC teams have worked with over 10,000 patients in more than 50 countries. We have 20 full-time practitioners and are considered one of the world's leading integrative medicine clinics. Along the way we've learnt a lot, and today we know infinitely more about fatigue-related conditions than I did back in the years when I was ill. Yet there is still so much more to be discovered; and, unfortunately for them, the greatest source of that learning is inevitably the patients who don't respond as we expect.

Our Journey Together

My aim in this book is to bring together the key principles of the approach I've developed alongside the OHC teams, to produce a practical guide that'll help you to help yourself. Although for many of you this won't necessarily replace the value of an online coaching program, or the need to work with a practitioner, there is a great deal you can do for yourself at home. Indeed, I'm deeply touched by the many comments I receive via email and social media from people who've been able to impact their healing journey dramatically by putting into action the tools you're about to learn, simply by following them online.

In setting the tone of this book, I intend to tread a number of delicate lines:

- I want to give you hope, without having you fall victim to the endless disappointment that I experienced.

- I aim to stay true to the scientific complexity of this group of conditions, while also making practical tools accessible to you.

- As my uncle did for me, I want to offer you compassion and empathy, while also being bold enough to give you a kick in the ass if and when you need it.

I'm sure that at times I'll fail in all of these intentions; however, I hope that by sharing them with you here, you'll at least know they're good! Furthermore, although this book is aimed at readers who are on a healing path from fatigue, I'm also aware that there are a number of medical experts who follow my work, and so, where appropriate, I've provided details of primary sources to assist those who wish to go deeper into the research that underpins our approach.

You may be reading this book as neither a sufferer nor a medical expert but as a caregiver or a relative of someone who's going through this immensely difficult experience, and so I've also included additional resources to support you.

I'm sad to say that my first-hand knowledge of fatigue isn't limited to my own experience and that of our patients – my sister-in-law suffered from chronic Lyme disease and at her most severe, she came to live with me and my wife for 2½ years; you'll read her story in the final chapter. Caring for her was its own unique challenge and as a result I can truly say that I've seen this group of conditions from every angle.

At this point I should also clarify that I loosely group the conditions chronic fatigue syndrome, myalgic encephalomyelitis, post-viral fatigue syndrome (including 'long COVID'), Lyme disease, fibromyalgia, and various others under the label 'fatigue-related conditions.' (I'll explain this further in the next few chapters.) I appreciate that this simplification is very far from perfect; however, as we'll discuss, while there are some unique defining features to some of these diagnoses, there are also unifying factors that make it helpful to talk about them together.

Lastly, you may be reading this as someone who's suffering from mild fatigue, and at times you might find my language a touch alarming, or even feel that it doesn't relate to your own experience – particularly when I describe instances in which people's entire lives are devastated by their symptoms. A helpful way to approach this is to consider that if these tools are effective even in those severe cases, they're highly likely to be helpful in much milder circumstances. Indeed, that's very much my experience.

The 12-Step Plan

At the heart of this book are 12 steps, or lessons, that'll not only help you to decode your fatigue but also to start to create your path to recovery and learn how best to navigate it. These are the same 12 steps that I look at with all of my patients at the OHC – and they form the core of our approach.

And guess what? We're already at the first of the 12 steps! Here's the thing: I know you didn't choose to have fatigue. What's more, you don't deserve it (no one does!) and you don't want it. And yet, whether you like it or not, right now it's happening and together we need to deal with it.

As my uncle helped me to realize, if you want the circumstances of your life to change, *you* have to be the one to change them. Indeed, that's our first step:

Step 1: Take responsibility

What I call radical responsibility means taking charge of our own life, on every level we can. Now, there is a very important distinction between blame and responsibility. You're not to blame for the situation in which you find yourself – you didn't do this deliberately – but if you don't take responsibility for changing it, the chances are that no one else will. So, before we go any further, I want to invite you to do the same exercise that my uncle set for me:

How Badly Do You Want Your Energy Back?

Take a few minutes to answer these questions and compile a list:

1. On a scale of 0–10, how badly do you want to get better?

2. Now make a list of all the things you know you could do to get better (you're going to learn a lot more in this book!)

3. How many hours a day do you spend doing the things that you've just identified as being helpful?

How to Use the Book

Right now, I challenge you to make a commitment to yourself: whatever it takes, at least finish this book. If you're struggling with motivation right now, I think you'll find that'll change if you stay with me in the coming pages. If you have the motivation but don't know where to start, that'll also, I hope, start to change.

In Part I, we're going to take the time to really understand what fatigue is, what causes it, and why conventional medicine has failed to truly understand it. In Part II, we're going to take the time to decode your fatigue together, and then in Part III we'll create a plan for your recovery.

You might feel tempted to jump straight to Parts II or III; however, because this book's content has been very carefully structured and it follows a particular sequence, I'd ask you to please read it in the order I've presented it. Also, just so you know, there are a few instances when I get a little technical; however, as this information isn't essential to your journey I've put it in boxes and you can skip it if you wish.

Finally, I've created a free online Decode Your Fatigue companion course to be used alongside this book. It includes video interviews with many of the people whose case studies you'll read in the coming chapters, along with quizzes and questionnaires to help bring further clarity, and even some recipe plans to help with my recommended dietary changes. You can access the course at www.alexhoward.com/fatigue.

Before we go any further, I think it's important to define what we actually mean when we refer to fatigue and fatigue-related conditions, and to explore why conventional medicine has likely failed you. So buckle up, and let's get stuck into the rather painful history of this complex but fascinating group of conditions.

■■ Chapter 2 ■■

WHY CONVENTIONAL MEDICINE IS BAFFLED BY FATIGUE

It was a freezing cold February morning and the first time I'd managed to get to school in over a month. Along with my fellow pupils, I'd returned after the Christmas holidays ready for another busy term, but just a week later, I'd experienced another severe crash of chronic fatigue. Even during one of my better periods, I could attend school for only a few hours a day, but one afternoon I'd done fractionally too much activity by trying to join an extra lesson and had then needed a month of recovery to get back to my pathetic baseline.

As I sat in the classroom waiting for the Economics lesson to begin, the usual feeling of loneliness kicked in. I'd never understood before how people can feel lonely when they're around others, but I found I no longer had anything in common with my classmates. I couldn't take part in sports, I rarely stayed for mealtimes, and I certainly couldn't attend any social events. I put on a brave face but often it was a struggle to even find anything to talk about.

It didn't help that I'd only been at this particular school for six months and hardly knew anyone because I'd missed so many lessons due to illness. One day a guy in my class asked me where I'd been. I explained by telling him I had chronic fatigue syndrome, and that I'd had a crash and had been resting in bed at home.

I can hear his response today as clearly as I did back then: 'You lucky git! Sounds like heaven to me! I wish I could spend a few weeks lying in bed and chilling out.'

I don't think my classmate intended to be unkind; at worst, his comment was a barbed joke, but it had a devastating effect on me. It was another nail in the coffin of my attempt to be understood by others, and I retreated a further step deeper into my own inner world.

Royal Free Disease

Almost two decades of working with others with fatigue in its varied and complex forms has taught me that I was far from alone in having experiences like this. In fact, I think one of the most difficult things about suffering from fatigue is the judgment and blame that seem to go along with it.

Fatigue and fatigue-related conditions such as myalgic encephalomyelitis (ME), chronic fatigue syndrome (CFS), and fibromyalgia are categorized as 'medically unexplained illnesses.' To be clear, this doesn't mean there are no explanations for them, only that *conventional medicine* is unable to explain them.[4, 5] Perhaps a more accurate label would be 'medically unexplained illnesses from a conventional medicine perspective.'

But why has conventional medicine failed so spectacularly to offer answers to those who are affected by fatigue? Given that understanding this question is the foundation of our entire adventure in decoding your fatigue, let's take some time to answer it. To do that, we need to take a step back in time, to 1950s Britain.

Between July and November 1955, 292 members of staff at London's Royal Free Hospital came down with a condition whose symptoms ranged from low-grade fever and swollen lymph nodes to severe headache and fatigue. Two hundred and fifty-five of those affected were admitted to the hospital, and by October it was forced to close temporarily to contain the outbreak. For many of these patients, symptoms went up and down over a long period, and in some cases their effects were devastating. And yet, despite considerable medical investigation and research, there was no identifiable cause of the outbreak.[6]

After the incident, Dr. Melvin Ramsay (of the Royal Free Hospital's infectious diseases department) coined the name myalgic encephalomyelitis for this condition, which means myalgic (muscle pain), encephalo (brain), myel (spinal cord), itis (inflammation),[7-9] to reflect the spinal cord inflammation in some of those affected, alongside the pain and headaches experienced.

With no medical explanation for myalgic encephalomyelitis, or Royal Free Disease, the hypothesis of mass hysteria was put forward, and to this day some pockets of medicine still refer to it as an example of collective medical hysteria with no physical origin.

The Legacy of Germ Theory

To understand why conventional medicine was so lost for answers in explaining the Royal Free outbreak, we need to take a further step back in the history books, to the formulation of a central belief of conventional medicine: germ theory.

Louis Pasteur was a 19th-century French chemist and microbiologist whose contribution to medical microbiology is almost without equal – among his discoveries were the principles of vaccination and microbial fermentation, and the food preparation process that bears his name, pasteurization. At the heart of Pasteur's impact was his evolution and popularization of germ theory, which is still accepted today.

The core tenet of germ theory is that the spread of microorganisms known as pathogens or 'germs' in the body can cause disease.[10, 11] Put in the simplest terms, from the common cold to the life-threatening sepsis, disease is the result of an external agent infecting the body and making us ill.

However, although Pasteur's germ theory wasn't fundamentally wrong, his work was incomplete. The problem with germ theory is that it perpetuates an over-simplified model of medicine that searches for a single cause, a test to measure it, and then a single drug to neutralize it or a vaccination to attempt to prevent it. That's fine when you're dealing with many acute illnesses, but it's a total disaster when you're seeking to understand multifaceted chronic illnesses.

As we'll soon discuss, fatigue is a complicated condition that has different subgroups, stages, and systems affected, each of which has its own unique signature in an individual sufferer. The application of germ theory to fatigue has failed at every juncture. After decades of searching, no one has managed to isolate a single pathogen, so there is no biomarker test and no uniform treatment in the form of a pharmaceutical drug.[12-15]

And, even when it comes to something seemingly clearly defined, such as 'long COVID' (i.e. fatigue symptoms that continue for 3–6 months after infection with coronavirus), the question still remains as to why some people recover within a few weeks, and others don't.

Aside from the devastating impact of the ineffectual application of germ theory to fatigue, and the resulting paralysis of research and treatment paths, I'd argue that there has also been an almost more severe consequence – the lack of a biomarker has resulted in the conclusion that fatigue must be 'all in the mind.'[16-18]

Arrogance on Steroids

Historically, the medical perspective on fatigue has been, 'We can't find anything wrong with you, so there isn't anything wrong with you.'

When you think about that statement from the fatigue patient's point of view, it's staggeringly arrogant. The inherent assumption is that conventional medicine knows everything there is to know about the human body, and because it can't find anything wrong with you, there *is* nothing wrong with you.

Indeed, in the decades following the Royal Free outbreak, the very limited research funding for fatigue went to the psychiatric community, to enable it to better understand the 'disordered thinking' of those with fatigue. The stories of personal tragedy that resulted from this approach lie beyond the focus of this book, but they're heartbreaking and enraging in equal measure.

If it hadn't been for the persistence and determination of an already vulnerable and depleted patient community, we'd probably still be stuck in the medical dark ages in our understanding of the nature of fatigue. We owe a lot to the brave, and at times truly heroic, actions of fatigue sufferers who have stood up for their rights and a deeper understanding of their experience.

In the last few decades endless lobbying and campaigning has resulted in full recognition of the validity of this group of chronic illnesses by the medical establishment. The USA's Centers for Disease Control (CDC) guidelines now say that 'myalgic encephalomyelitis/chronic fatigue syndrome (ME/CFS) is a serious, long-term illness that affects many body systems.'[19]

Progress has undoubtedly been made, but unfortunately, it's done little to cure the arrogance of conventional medicine. Common medical understanding has moved from 'We can't find anything wrong with you, so there is nothing wrong with you' to 'Clearly there *is* something wrong with you, but we don't have any answers. So there *are* no answers.'

Think about that for a moment. Once again, the inherent assumption is that conventional medicine has all the answers: 'We don't understand what's happening, and therefore it's either not real or it's not possible to understand it.' This isn't just arrogance – it's arrogance on steroids.

Now at this point you'd be forgiven for thinking that I harbor ill will toward the medical establishment for what is at best incompetence, and at worst abuse, toward fatigue sufferers. But in fact, you'd be wrong. Conventional medicine saves countless lives every day – we only have to look at the incredible work done by our healthcare systems in response to COVID-19 to see this. And if I get knocked down by a bus, you won't hear me screaming for a nutritionist and a psychotherapist – no, I want the painkillers, the surgeon, and whatever else modern medicine can offer to save my life.

So I'm not opposed to conventional medicine – I'm just against arrogance and closed minds. And, unfortunately, there is quite a bit of that around in both conventional and non-conventional medical circles. Of course, when we're dealing with life, death, and intense human suffering on a daily basis, it's understandable that we need to have a certain confidence in our approach. Imagine being the pilot of an airliner with hundreds of trusting passengers, and each step of the journey questioning whether the plane will stay in the air, whether you have what it takes to fly it, whether the engines are going to work, and so on. You'd go crazy before the first day was over.

Certainty is a reasonable human need, and maintaining a curious, open, and discerning mind is no easy feat when working as a medical practitioner. Yes, it's a very big thing to ask of our physicians; and yet, it's also critical when faced with complex and deeply misunderstood conditions such as fatigue.

Indeed, during my conversations with GP friends over the years, many have told me that they feel something similar. The truth is that most doctors dread seeing patients with chronic illnesses they don't understand.[20, 21] At the end of the day, your typical doctor chooses a career in medicine because they want to help people, and after years of physically, emotionally, and mentally grueling training, the last thing they want is to sit across from patients who are suffering and feel powerless to help them.

The coldness and harshness that patient communities feel from their GPs isn't a reflection of their lack of caring – instead, it's a defensive strategy that doctors use to avoid feeling their sense of inadequacy and failure.[22]

A New Paradigm for Medicine

So, given the fundamental problems with a conventional medical approach to working with fatigue, you can begin to see why sufferers face such an uphill battle to find answers and to decode their fatigue.

But, as always, where there is a problem, there is an opportunity, and over the years there have been a number of trailblazers looking for answers. Some have been seen as rebels, some as outcasts, and others have managed to cruise below the radar while doing outstanding and important work.

The terms 'alternative' and 'complementary' medicine have become popular in recent years, but personally I don't like either of them; I think they imply that non-conventional methods are somehow lesser than those of conventional medicine and need to be kept on the side. I prefer the term integrative medicine [23, 24] because I believe a truly holistic approach will integrate anything that has relevance to supporting the healing journey.

In more recent years, the concept of functional medicine has been gathering recognition,[25] and indeed, I feel it best captures the essence of the approach we use at The Optimum Health Clinic. Functional medicine 'employs a systems-oriented medical approach that works to identify and understand the underlying or root causes of a disease.' Put another way, rather than treating symptoms, in functional medicine we're really looking to dive deeper into the root causes of your fatigue.

Defining Fatigue

In that spirit, before we go any further, we need to define exactly what we're talking about when we speak of fatigue. In the dictionary, fatigue is defined as 'extreme tiredness resulting from mental or physical exertion or illness.' However, I'm not sure how helpful this is.

If your levels of mental or physical exertion are excessive, then your fatigue doesn't require decoding and your remedy is simple: live a more balanced life. What's more likely is that your levels of exertion are normal and yet you still experience fatigue. This leaves us with the real question – *why* does a normal level of activity leave you fatigued?

Perhaps you've just recently started to find that the day is longer than the energy you have to meet it, and that your afternoon energy dip is no longer defeated by a strong espresso. Perhaps you've suffered with severe fatigue for many years, or maybe you've oscillated between phases of normal functioning and phases of fatigue but have never felt that your energy is reliable in the way it should be.

Regardless, the reason you're reading this book is that something remains unexplained. You aren't just a mystery to modern medicine – you're a mystery to yourself. And it's my hope that by the time you reach the end of this book, that mystery will be solved, at least in part.

Diagnosing Fatigue

This brings us to the second step in our 12-step plan:

Step 2: Get an accurate diagnosis

You see, a diagnosis of fatigue is no diagnosis at all: fatigue is a *symptom*, not a condition in itself. The reason we need to decode your fatigue is that fatigue, whether it's self-diagnosed or medically diagnosed, is ultimately a false diagnosis. To really understand this point, we need to explore the diagnostic process for fatigue-related conditions.

A diagnosis of fatigue isn't a diagnosis of the presence of a particular physical injury, a particular pathogen, or even a specific marker or set of markers that are out of balance. A diagnosis of fatigue, be it chronic or otherwise, is a diagnosis of exclusion. That means it's a diagnosis in the absence of any known cause.

The Diagnostic Process

The diagnostic process for fatigue should go something like this.

1. You go to your doctor because you feel exhausted, and perhaps have some other symptoms such as muscle pain, dizziness, or sleep issues.

2. Your doctor considers your symptoms and history and orders a standard set of blood tests that look at basic markers such as full blood cell count; iron and ferritin levels; the inflammation markers ESR or CRP; liver, kidney, and thyroid function; tests for diabetes, and a celiac screen. Ideally, this will also include Vitamin D and what's called a bone profile, and a test to rule out glandular fever.[26, 27]

3. The doctor will also investigate any other abnormalities that could explain the fatigue you're experiencing. The purpose of this is to rule out various other explanations, such as autoimmune disease, thyroid, and more rarely, cardiac or pituitary disease, sleep disorders, neurodegenerative disease, diabetes, or some cancers.[28]

4. If those investigations come back abnormal in any way your doctor will do further investigations and potentially refer you to a specialist consultant, resulting in a different diagnosis.

5. If the markers all come back normal, or, following the referral there is no known cause and no other obvious reason for your fatigue,

you'll get a diagnosis of a 'fatigue-related condition' such as chronic fatigue syndrome, fibromyalgia, or post-viral fatigue syndrome.[29, 30]

Now, there is a *very* important point being made in the above process. If you're suffering with fatigue, chronic or otherwise, it's of critical importance that you engage with a suitably qualified medical professional to thoroughly investigate the conventional medical approach. There are multiple causes of fatigue that are identifiable by orthodox medicine,[28, 31, 32] and if any of these is the culprit, acting sooner rather than later could literally be the difference between life and death.

So please, before you go any further in this book, make sure you've been fully assessed by a suitably qualified medical doctor and that you've gone through the steps above; or at the very least, do it in parallel (unless your doctor is willing to follow a number of lines of investigation at the same time, this process can take many months.) Don't take this warning lightly, and don't delay or put off seeing a doctor.

That said, going forward, I'm assuming that you've engaged with a suitable medical professional and the problem is that they couldn't decode your fatigue, despite having followed medical due process. If this has happened, the good news is that there is unlikely to be anything life-threatening underlying your symptoms, which means we can get to work on decoding your fatigue together and creating your path toward healing.

At this point, you'd be excused for thinking, *Well Alex, I've already had a diagnosis of chronic fatigue syndrome, so all of the above doesn't apply to me.* Actually, I disagree. A diagnosis of chronic fatigue syndrome really just means that your fatigue is 'chronic,' otherwise known as ongoing. Adding the word syndrome might make it sound more official, but it tells us nothing further about what's actually going on.

There is also so much disparity in the definition, diagnosis, and treatment of chronic fatigue[33] that although it can be a relief to have a name for what's happening, it may not get you very much further with your healing. In fact, as controversial as it might sound, I have a similar attitude to diagnoses such as post-viral fatigue syndrome, myalgic encephalomyelitis, and fibromyalgia – none of these is actually a helpful diagnosis.

A useful medical diagnosis would be something like, 'You've torn your ACL ligament' or 'You have appendicitis.' Of course, my point isn't that you'd want either of these diagnoses, but they would at least be accurate and give you a clear path toward treatment.

How about fibromyalgia, you might ask. Well, fibromyalgia is another condition with its own history of controversy,[33, 34] but in essence we're still talking about a fatigue condition, except with the additional symptom of pain.

And what about Lyme disease and coinfections? As we'll get into in Chapter 11, we're at least closer here to a helpful diagnosis; however, as many people with chronic Lyme disease have experienced, using a typical germ theory approach of nuking the Lyme disease is rarely as effective as one might hope.[35-39] We still need to look at a multisystem approach and take into account more than just the immune system and its inability to fight the Lyme.

Although it can be unsettling to step free of the certainty of a medical diagnosis, I believe it's also deeply empowering. By diving deeper into understanding what's truly going on for you, you're a step closer to decoding your fatigue and plotting your path to recovery. And, although this will be an intricate and challenging path, when you start to find real answers, it'll also become an exciting one.

Before we move on, we need to get super clear on something: the exact biochemical process behind fatigue. What's actually going on at a cellular level? What would you say if I told you that we can answer this question with great specificity? You see, in fact, your fatigue is likely very far from being medically unexplained – a very well understood biochemical process is causing it.

■■ Chapter 3 ■■

HOW YOUR BODY CREATES ENERGY

It was an early evening in the autumn of 2005 and I was about to head home from work. However experienced you become as a practitioner, seeing patients one after the other throughout the day is mentally and emotionally demanding, and the last thing I felt like right then was a long conversation about complex cellular biology.

In those days, The Optimum Health Clinic was located in a basement on London's Harley Street; it wasn't quite as glamorous as it sounds, but it was a huge step up from the bedsit in which we'd started. As I closed my laptop and began to pack up my things, I felt that sense of satisfaction you get after a hard day's work done well. I was ready to leave when Niki Gratrix, my cofounder, burst into my clinic room. She had a look of frantic excitement in her eyes, which I knew meant I wasn't going home anytime soon.

'Alex, you're not going to believe what I've been reading about today,' she began. One of the things that I most loved about working with Niki was her intense passion and excitement for learning, and at times like this it was infectious.

'Alex, seriously – this is the most important breakthrough in fatigue research I've come across. I'm telling you, this is going to change everything,' she continued.

I took a deep breath, waved goodbye to my lazy evening on the sofa, and replied: 'OK, that's some big talk. What is it?'

'So, what's the biggest outstanding mystery of fatigue?' Niki asked with an expectant look on her face.

I was tempted to say something facetious, like: 'I don't know – why is being tired so tiring?' But making fun of Niki in that moment would have been a bit like shooting an excited puppy, so instead, I played along: 'I don't know, you tell me,' I said.

'Post-exertional malaise,' Niki continued. 'Why is it that someone with fatigue can have the energy to do something and then their energy crashes afterward?'

Niki had sparked my curiosity there – she certainly had a point. It was bad enough that people with fatigue had low energy in the first place, but it never seemed to make sense that they could do something at the time, and then afterward, crash for no obvious reason. Post-exertional malaise (PEM), as this is known, is not only one of the most mysterious symptoms of chronic fatigue but also one of the most deeply frustrating and painful for sufferers.

'OK, you've got my attention,' I said. 'If you can explain why that happens, and more importantly, tell me that you have some kind of solution and you aren't exaggerating, then this is a big deal.'

Over the next hour or so, Niki patiently outlined to me the groundbreaking research she'd seen on ATP and mitochondrial function.[40] For the first time, someone was able to explain to me not only the actual mechanism of low energy but also why people with fatigue will crash, seemingly out of nowhere.

What Is Energy?

Before we can fully explore what Niki explained to me, there is a fundamental question we need to answer – if fatigue is the absence of energy, what actually is energy? What is this mysterious currency that's in such short supply when someone feels fatigue?

Let's think about currency for a moment. It's a means of exchange that allows something to move around – as in the way we use money to exchange goods in trade. The energy currency of your body is an energy-rich molecule called adenosine triphosphate, or ATP for short. ATP provides the fuel for pretty much every function in your body that requires energy – from nerve cell impulses to muscle cell contraction to fueling your brain, your heart and all the other organs of the body. Ultimately, the energy source keeping your body alive is ATP.

So, if ATP is the currency of energy in the body, it seems reasonable to assume that endurance-trained athletes have higher levels of ATP at rest, and are better at making it when demanded by exercise. And this is very much the case. A study published in 2018 found that when compared to controls, trained athletes demonstrate 10 percent more ATP at rest and possess significantly increased levels of ATP during exercise activity.[41]

Furthermore, trained athletes have the ability to increase available ATP by 100 percent more than controls during exercise. Put simply, the factor that allows endurance athletes to perform at the levels they do is that they're literally making more energy currency.

Where Does Energy Come From?

If ATP is the currency of energy in our body, we now have another, equally important, question to answer – where does our energy come from? What's the process by which the body makes energy? And why is it that an endurance athlete appears to have energy in abundance and yet someone with fatigue has to ration their energy, as though supplies might run out at any moment?

Well, ATP is manufactured by specialized structures inside our cells called mitochondria. If ATP is the currency of energy, the mitochondria are the energy factories that make the currency – they are effectively the 'powerhouses' of the cell. Almost all living cells have mitochondria; some cells produce more than others, but every single cell in your body, apart from red blood cells, has its own powerhouse. Indeed, fat cells have many mitochondria because they store energy, and equally, muscle cells have a lot because they need to respond quickly to energy demand.

At this point, you're likely thinking, *Well, to decode my fatigue, I just need to get my mitochondria working properly.* And in a sense you're right. This is the next step in our 12-step plan:

Step 3: Understand the role of your mitochondria

Essentially, our mitochondria help turn the energy we take from food into energy that the cell can use. The actual chemical process of how they do this is pretty long-winded, and you don't need a full understanding of it in order for us to continue our journey together; however, for those of you who remember some of your high-school biochemistry, the following technical box may serve as a helpful summary. (As I explained in Chapter 1, these boxes are optional rather than critical.)

▪▪ How Our Mitochondria Make Energy ▪▪

Energy production in the mitochondria begins with the food we eat. Plants use photosynthesis to capture energy from light in the form of carbohydrates, and humans obtain that stored energy by digesting and absorbing it – either directly from plants or from the animals that consume them (we'll get into your digestion in Chapter 9).

Your mitochondria combine these molecules from food with oxygen and convert them to water and carbon dioxide, releasing energy. This process is called aerobic respiration.

The energy produced through aerobic respiration is stored within the energy-carrying molecule ATP (adenosine triphosphate). ATP has three (tri') phosphate groups, linked to each other by bonds (see top of diagram). The energy is trapped in the bonds to each phosphate group and in that way it can be transported to where it's needed.

Energy is released when the bond between the second and third phosphate group is broken. The remaining molecule (having released one phosphate group) becomes adenosine diphosphate, or ADP.

ADP can then be transported back into the mitochondria and recharged into ATP through chemical reactions that add the third phosphate molecule back (see center of diagram). This is known as ADP/ATP 'recycling' and is the most efficient way to generate new energy. When any aspect of this process isn't working effectively, we'll experience post-exertional malaise.

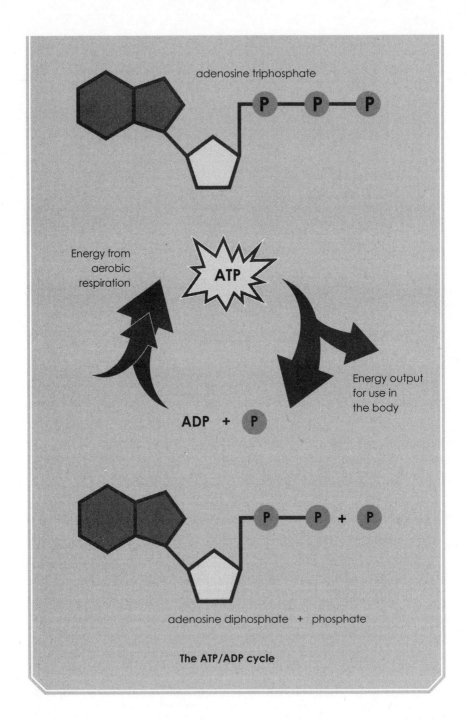

adenosine triphosphate

Energy from aerobic respiration

ATP

Energy output for use in the body

ADP + P

adenosine diphosphate + phosphate

The ATP/ADP cycle

Post-Exertional Malaise Explained

So, now that we've discussed the basic principles behind what energy is and how it's created, let's return to my crucial conversation with Niki. As I mentioned earlier, one of the most frustrating symptoms of fatigue is post-exertional malaise (PEM), and also what we call the 'delayed fatigue response,' which is when the fatigue takes several days to appear; more on this in a moment.

After a lie-down or a good night's sleep, a healthy individual can expect to feel the same as they did before a modest level of exertion, but this isn't the case with ongoing fatigue. Let's say you're struggling with low energy but are just about managing to function at a low level. It's Saturday afternoon, you have friends visiting, and everyone decides to go for a walk. Now, this walk is a stretch on what you'd do on an average day but you don't want to let people down – and actually, you feel like getting some fresh air.

Over the next couple of hours, you maintain a steady pace and walk around three or four miles. It's been a while since you blew away the cobwebs like this, and you find you're having a better time than you expected. That evening your muscles are a bit stiff, but you go to bed feeling relieved that you got through it – and a little surprised that you're not paying more of a price.

On Sunday morning your body still feels a little stiff, but you seem fine. You notice that your nervous system is perhaps a little overstimulated and that you're finding it difficult to take it easy. Maybe yesterday's walk has given you some more energy.

When you wake up for work on Monday morning you feel as if you've been hit by a train. You're utterly exhausted. You feel faint simply standing up, all your muscles hurt, and with little choice, you call in sick. Your symptoms don't improve for a few days – you continue to feel totally wiped out – before gradually getting better.

You find yourself wondering, *What the heck just happened?* It must have been the walk – but why did it take several days before you felt the impact, and why did it then take several days for you to recover?

This is the delayed fatigue response, and it's a key feature of many people's fatigue. They do something and they seem OK, and it's only several days later that they feel the impact of it; for others, there isn't even a delay – whenever they go beyond their energy capacity, there is a resulting exhaustion. This is what's technically known as post-exertional malaise (PEM).

PEM is a well-documented factor in chronic fatigue syndrome.[42, 43] A 2010 study of 48 women with CFS found that 60 percent of them took five days to feel better after exertion.[44] And it's not only exercise that causes PEM[45] – it can also have physical and physiological,[46, 47] emotional,[48] cognitive,[49, 50] or sensory and environmental causes.[45, 51]

So, what's the relationship between mitochondrial function, ATP, and PEM? Well, it's all down to how ATP is generated within your mitochondria. Here's another technical explanation for those of you who are interested.

■■ ATP Recycling and ■■ Post-Exertional Malaise

Each of our mitochondria has the capacity to produce 36–48 ATP (units of energy) from scratch. This is a lengthy biochemical process that can take up to two days. The majority of our energy (ATP) production is needed 'on demand' when we use it for cellular activities such as exercise, so instead of making it all from scratch, we take a shortcut by *recycling* the ADP we produced earlier. This process, which takes about 10 seconds, is called oxidative phosphorylation, and it's responsible for meeting about 60 percent of our energy demand.

Oxidative phosphorylation is responsive to the needs of our body, and with normal mitochondrial functioning, we can train our body to become more efficient and produce more energy. As long as we don't over-train the body, the more demand it gets used to, the better this process of oxidative phosphorylation is able to work, including making more mitochondria. Remember what we discussed earlier about endurance athletes?

However, in certain situations when this recycling isn't taking place quickly enough to meet demand, two ADPs can be combined to form one ATP and one adenosine monophosphate (AMP), releasing only a small amount of energy. In muscle, AMP may be further broken down to inosine monophosphate (IMP), which may then be lost altogether through the urine.

Making ATP from AMP is a very slow and energy-consuming process, and it takes some days for the body to recharge, particularly if AMP has been depleted. This is why we can end up experiencing post-exertional malaise.

Put simply, the cause of fatigue is suboptimal, or inefficient, ATP recycling. If we push ourselves beyond our capacity, ADP is converted to AMP, which can only be recycled much more slowly. It then takes several days to make fresh ATP from new raw ingredients. Ultimately, fatigue is the result of not having enough ATP or ADP from which adequate levels of energy can be made.

Here's the thing – you're not crazy: your fatigue is real. There is a very clear and specific process in your body that's likely not working properly. And guess what? We can even test it.

Testing Mitochondrial Function

In the days following Niki's initial discoveries we were even more excited to discover that a UK-based laboratory was pioneering mitochondrial function testing in fatigue patients. Dr. John McLaren Howard was collaborating with Dr. Sarah Myhill, one of the British pioneers of functional medicine for fatigue patients, and they'd developed a truly groundbreaking blood test.[52, 53]

In addition to rating how efficiently a patient's mitochondria produced energy, this test could also look for possible issues with toxicity and blockages of the mitochondria. Niki and I quickly realized the test could be a big advantage when working with our patients. There was, however, a rather major hurdle – the laboratory would only work directly with medics, and at this point there were no doctors working in the OHC practitioner team.

Undeterred, I got straight on the phone to a medic friend and asked them if they'd be willing to sponsor all of our mitochondrial testing with the laboratory, which they were more than happy to do. And, over time, due to the sheer volume of testing we were doing, we forged our own relationship with a further lab internationally offering such tests. In the years since then, we've performed thousands of mitochondrial function tests, and we've found it to be an enormously useful clinical tool.

The beauty of testing mitochondrial function is that we have the ability to break down the complicated business of making energy into a series of logical steps and physiological questions. And, having conducted so many tests over the years, the learning is enormously important in making sense of a patient's clinical picture, even when we don't test. For the patient, this information is invariably the first time that anyone has been able to explain the physiology behind their fatigue, and as such it's often met with great excitement and at times, huge emotion.

Fueling the Mitochondria

Now, you can probably guess what happened next. Inspired by the outstanding work of others in the field, we'd discovered how energy is created, and we also knew which raw ingredients the body uses to make energy. What was the obvious conclusion to come to? You've guessed it – we decided to start supplementing those patients with poor mitochondrial function with these raw ingredients!

Using carefully designed protocols of supplements such as co-enyzme Q-10, D-ribose, magnesium, and L-carnitine,[54, 55] we dosed people up to see what would happen. The results? In some cases, they were astounding. For some patients it was almost like a miracle. People who'd struggled with severe fatigue for years literally felt as if someone had plugged their body back into the mains circuit again. Patients who felt as if they'd tried everything to combat their fatigue suddenly had an explanation for the symptoms and a test demonstrating what was wrong; and they also had an effective strategy to correct it. It was almost like germ theory at its finest.

Unfortunately, although those miracle cases can still happen, and using appropriate raw ingredients to support mitochondrial function is still part of our wider approach for some patients, experience has shown us that it's often not that simple.

Fueling the mitochondria with raw ingredients can be a bit like pouring more fuel into a faulty engine. We noticed that some people ended up with a lot more energy with which to return to their former life, but they eventually crashed again, this time more severely and further, therefore compounding the issue. Others found they were more wired with energy but were unable to sleep, and their other symptoms ended up worse rather than better.

Part of mitigating these issues was about dosing and going slowly with supplements. However, we also came to realize a much more important truth – in many cases, fatigue isn't healed by treating the mitochondria directly. Mitochondrial malfunction may often be the culmination of the perfect storm of functional deficiencies and burdens further upstream. So, ultimately, to decode the puzzle of your fatigue, we need to trace a pathway backward from the mitochondria.

Indeed, as I reflect on that conversation with Niki in those early years of our work, I realize it was just as critical as I thought at the time, but for a different reason: by understanding the mechanisms of fatigue, we can better target everything else we're doing at the clinic, and we understand on an even deeper level why our interventions work.

In fact, as you'll discover in Chapter 5, there are a number of factors that affect mitochondrial function, and it's by addressing and balancing these that your body is able to heal. And, as you're about to discover, one of the most powerful ways of changing our mitochondria is shifting what's happening in our nervous system.

You see, rather sneakily, in this chapter I haven't mentioned another vital role of your mitochondria, which may well be the key to unlocking your healing. We're going to explore how the mind–body connection has a direct impact on your energy production.

■■ Chapter 4 ■■

HOW YOUR MIND AND EMOTIONS AFFECT FATIGUE

Nick was in his mid-thirties and had been a police officer since leaving school. It was a career he loved and his ambition had taken him a long way. In his most recent assignment, he'd undertaken the highest level of undercover work the police do, and he'd felt privileged and proud to be chosen.

Within a few months of Nick starting this two-year assignment, his sergeant had a stroke, a colleague was killed in the line of duty, and his closest police partner was diagnosed with a mental illness stemming from the problems and pressures of the job. However, Nick's attitude to stress at the time was that 'it was just being busy.' He described the police force as an environment in which 'you kick on, you kick through, and you maintain professionalism in your image.'

'I wanted to maintain my part in it,' he explained to me. 'Selfish or not, there is this image that we cops want to keep, and mine was of this burly copper who ain't going down, who isn't going to show any emotion, and has to get on with it.'

For the duration of Nick's undercover assignment there was no support for him and the difficult emotions he was experiencing – not only due to the loss of his colleagues but also the dangerous and intense work he was doing. Throughout the assignment, Nick had seemed fine, but within a month of completing it he started to develop symptoms of fatigue and muscle pains. Things went from bad to worse, and in time he was forced to stop working completely and was diagnosed with ME/CFS.

Nick then came across my first book, *Why Me? My Journey From ME to Health and Happiness*, and, inspired by my belief that it's possible to recover, he came to see us at the OHC; he worked with me on the psychology side and with one of our nutritional therapists on the physical side. Nick had no lack of commitment and determination to get well but he was also honest about the fact he was deeply skeptical that talking about his thoughts and feelings would have any impact on his physical body.

As he sat on the train home from his first consultation with me, Nick decided the trip had been a waste of time. 'At the time I wasn't open enough,' he later told me. 'I wasn't open to what I was being told and I probably wasn't ready to receive and embrace it. I believed that if you got sick, you took a pill and you got better. I wanted the pill; I wanted the GP to say, "There is your ME pill. Swallow it and you'll be all right on Monday."'

However, Nick did follow to the letter the nutritional advice he was given, and he couldn't deny that it had a fairly immediate and significant impact on his energy levels. Realizing that he needed more persuading about the role of psychology, I put him in touch with a former patient called Colin (whose story you'll read in Chapter 8), who shared his experience of the direct and immediate impact of working with his psychology.

Nick returned to the clinic for further psychology sessions with a more curious attitude, and together we did some good work, following an early version of the approach you're about to learn. Nick would later say, 'I would never have spoken a few years ago about the connection between mind and body. This has been a massive transformation for me in many ways. The change has been internal rather than external. You have to get yourself in the environment internally and externally where you're going to heal.'

Nick went on to make a full recovery and returned to his career with the police force, where he remains to this day. If Nick, a 'burly copper who ain't going down,' can learn to understand his thoughts and feelings and work with them to support his healing, then I think it's possible for anyone to do so.

The Role of Psychology

As I'd explained to Nick, there is an awkward truth with many chronic illnesses. Whether we like it or not, psychology plays a critical role in healing. I know this may not be what you want to hear, and I know that when the same was said to me it felt deeply offensive – the inference was that there was nothing wrong me and I was making up the hell I was living in. But if you can just hang in there with me, I want to make a few important points.

When we speak of the role of psychology, we're not talking about fatigue being 'in the mind.' In fact, it's quite the opposite – as we'll get into – fatigue is very much in the body. When people think of something as being 'in the mind,' the inherent assumption is that it's not real. An example of this is phantom limb pain – someone's tragically lost a limb and yet they continue to experience pain in that limb, as if it still exists. As real as their pain might be, it's in their mind (albeit unconsciously) not their body. As we saw in the previous section, the same cannot be said of fatigue.

Another perception of something being 'in the mind' is that it's just a lack of motivation, a form of depression. The conclusion therefore is that if one can just 'get motivated' or 'have something exciting to look forward to,' then somehow the symptoms will abate. If only it were that simple.

Although depression is a real and difficult experience in itself, its fundamental biochemistry is very different from that of fatigue, as is the pathway to recovery.[56-58] The felt experience of depression is that all we want to do is climb into bed and hide away from the world. With fatigue it's the opposite – all we want to do is climb out of bed and come back into the world, but we simply don't have the energy to do it.

Misdiagnosing fatigue as depression is a serious error. Whereas the research on depression clearly demonstrates that exercise and a certain level of social interaction are beneficial,[59-62] the findings on fatigue are the direct opposite.[63-66] I should also state that depression can sometimes be an inevitable consequence of suffering from fatigue; however, in that instance it's a *symptom* of fatigue,[67] not the *cause* of it.

The Origins of Mind–body Medicine

The fact that our mind affects our body isn't a controversial one. Indeed, anyone who's salivated in anticipation of a favorite meal (i.e. their body responds to the food before they've eaten it) will struggle to deny that what we think can make things happen in our body. However, the science of just how powerfully and deeply our mind and body are connected is only just getting started.

In 1986, a landmark study published by Dr. Janice Kiecolt-Glaser and her colleagues demonstrated the impact of stress on the immune system.[68] The researcher team took blood samples from 34 medical students one month before their examinations and a second on the day of the exams. On exam day, there were significant declines in a number of measures, including the activity of natural killer (NK) cells, whose job it is to contain and help kill infections. Ultimately, stress led to a reduced ability to fight infections and a greater likelihood of becoming ill.

Another important paper, published in 2011, collated data from a number of studies over the years demonstrating the impact of psychological stress on wound healing.[69] To quote the authors, 'Psychological stress can have a substantial and clinically relevant effect on wound repair.'

The paper gives multiple examples of a number of different ways of assessing the impact of stress on wound healing, but I think one of the most interesting is the first study, conducted in 1995, which involved family caregivers to those suffering from dementia.[70] The daily stress of living with loved ones' loss of memory, inappropriate emotions, and wandering and restless behavior is considerable. Indeed, caregiving stress has been associated with heightened anxiety and depression, immune dysregulation, an increased risk for cardiovascular disorders, and even death.

A 3.5 mm punch biopsy wound was created on the nondominant forearm of 13 women who were caring for relatives with dementia and 13 non-caregiving controls who were similar in demographics and makeup. The researchers found that the wound took 24 percent longer to heal in the caregivers than in the controls. Put simply, stress slows down the body's healing capacity.

How Stress Affects Energy Production

As I outlined at the start of this chapter, it's very common to feel both cynical about and resistant to the idea that psychology plays an important role in fatigue. And yet, as we've been exploring, there is undeniable evidence that our mind has an impact on our body. But the relationship between stress and energy isn't only an indirect one; in fact, stress directly impacts our energy production.

Back in 2008, we had a patient called Louise who lived in Singapore and was suffering from quite severe ME/CFS. Keen to make progress as quickly as possible, she was working with our nutrition and psychology teams in tandem.

To help us get as deep an understanding as possible of what was going on for Louise, we decided to do mitochondrial testing to explore how well her body was producing and recycling energy on a cellular level. However, the only lab offering this at the time was based in London, so there were some logistical challenges, to say the least, in getting samples halfway across the world before they degraded.

At one point it appeared that Louise's samples had been lost in the mail, and so she focused on working with our psychology team to calm her nervous system and cultivate a healing state in her body. As a result of various delays, including Louise's family holidays, it was three months before we could arrange for a replacement test kit to be sent to Singapore, the samples returned, and the results analyzed.

We then discovered that Louise's original test kit *had* been analyzed and it was the results that had been misplaced. So we found ourselves with two test results, with the only intervention between them being a strong focus on our psychology approach.

The results were pretty astounding. There'd been a dramatic improvement in Louise's mitochondrial function, and, given that she'd been ill for several years without improvement, this was unlikely to be a coincidence. Calming her nervous system had directly impacted her mitochondrial function.

Cell Danger Response

At the clinic we'd become used to seeing a patient's energy transformed as a result of calming their nervous system; however, it would be another decade before I came across the science that truly explained cases such as Louise's. Put another way – we knew what we did worked but this finding could finally explain the actual biology.

Dr. Robert Naviaux is a professor in residence at the University of California in San Diego, and at the heart of his work is the idea that the human body is a highly intelligent system that's evolved through millennia to protect its own survival under stress. His theory is called cell danger response (CDR), and it explains how our cells act differently when we're under extreme and prolonged stress.[71, 72]

Dr. Naviaux says that: 'The cell danger response (CDR) is the evolutionarily conserved metabolic response that protects cells and hosts from harm. It's triggered by encounters with chemical, physical, or biological threats that exceed the cellular capacity for homeostasis [the process by which biological systems maintain an internal stability that persists despite conditions in the world outside]'.[71]

Later, we'll get much more into the concept of stress, and how suffering from fatigue is in itself a trigger for stress, as well as a consequence of it, but first, I want to explore further the impact of stress on our actual cellular energy production.

When we talked about mitochondria in the last chapter, I didn't tell you the whole story. While our mitochondria are the powerhouses of our cellular energy production, they also have a second, equally important, job – danger signaling. They are the body's equivalent of the canary in the coalmine.

Coal miners face many dangers, one of which is the risk of death from gases such as methane and carbon dioxide. In the old days, miners would take a canary in a cage down with them to provide an early warning mechanism. If there were dangerous levels of these colorless, odorless gases in the mine, the canary would fall unconscious, signaling to the miners that they needed to get out of the mine immediately. Indeed, my paternal grandfather was a coal miner, so I may well owe my very existence to the effectiveness of those canaries and their early warning system.

Our mitochondria have the same function in our body. Because their metabolism is so fast, they are the first to sense danger or toxicity; in fact, although inside the cell the focus of the mitochondria is their work as an energy carrier metabolism, outside the cell they have a completely different role as a signaling molecule that warns neighboring cells if there is stress in the environment.

But here's the really important thing: when the cell danger response (CDR) is activated, the mitochondria switch their priorities. They de-prioritize energy production in order to free up resources to prioritize danger signaling.[73] Put simply, when your body's under stress, you make less energy so your body can protect itself.

For the first time, thanks to Dr. Naviaux's emerging paradigm-shifting work, we can explain a great many cases like Louise's. When we calm the nervous system, the body enters a healing state and can re-prioritize energy production. In other words, when your body is calmer, you get more energy.

In Parts II and III of the book, we're going to get much further into what causes stress in the nervous system, and how to cultivate a healing state. But for now, it's critical you understand that the mind–body connection isn't just some theory – it's a very real factor in decoding and healing your fatigue.

So, now that we've explored how your body creates energy and the critical role of mind–body medicine, we have enough of the foundations to get into the model of fatigue I've spent the last quarter of a century creating.

Chapter 5

A NEW MODEL FOR
UNDERSTANDING FATIGUE

I remember the feeling as if it happened yesterday... I was eight years old and standing at the counter of a hiking shop, about to buy a compass. It felt just like Christmas morning, and I was full of anticipation and excitement.

My mother had recently remarried, and my stepfather loved walking. I'd not had a father figure for the previous seven years, so that meant I too loved walking and everything that went with it. I'd been saving up my pocket money for months to buy this compass: a seemingly magical device that would reliably show the way.

This was the late 1980s – long before a compass became just one of thousands of apps we have at our disposal, let alone Google maps, making such a tool seem utterly primitive. When I got home, the first thing I did was pull out the map of our local area from my stepfather's cherished map collection. With a little bit of guidance, I could now direct myself around the neighborhood with confidence. In fact, as long as I had my compass and the correct map, I could navigate anywhere.

A decade or so later – soon after that fateful conversation with my uncle – I found myself thinking about that compass and those maps. Here I was on the most challenging voyage of my life, and I had no map and no compass. Motivation and discipline alone were not enough – if I was going to have any chance of escaping my illness, I needed a map.

Mapping Your Fatigue

Much of the next seven years of my life was about creating my own map of fatigue, through a painful and frustrating process of trial and error. Each twist and turn had its own story, and its own painful experience, that helped me navigate it better next time around.

Sitting here writing this book, several more decades later, I'm immensely proud of the map that's been created through my own experiences of fatigue and those of the tens of thousands of people we've supported at the OHC.

But it's been far from an easy process. We're enormously indebted to all the patients we've worked with over the years at the OHC, each of whom, in their own way, has helped us to confirm elements of the map – or indeed to discover its limitations – and day by day, patient by patient, it has evolved and improved.

As we explore the fatigue map together, I guarantee that you'll find limitations and places where it doesn't match your own experience. This is partly because the map is imperfect and partly because for the sake of brevity, I've had to shorten it drastically in places. Indeed, the value of a map lies in its ability to simplify something complicated to help us navigate more efficiently – by definition, nuances and details are left out, and there are always exceptions to every rule.

That said, I've yet to meet a patient for whom at least some elements of this map were not immensely useful in decoding their fatigue, and for many people it's like going from seeing the world in black and white to seeing it in color for the first time.

In this chapter, my aim is to introduce you to the fatigue map – which we use every day in the clinic and with every client. It has two parts: map 1, which helps us understand how you got ill in the first place, and map 2, which helps us understand the key stages of your path to recovery.

Fatigue Map 1: Understanding How You've Become Fatigued

Let's start by briefly exploring map 1. As we've discussed, your fatigue is multifaceted and is impacted by a number of factors. You have your underlying genetics, which create certain vulnerabilities; you then have your personality and the way you approach your life; and on top of this, you have the various loads, or traumas, that have impacted you in your lifetime.

These factors, together, result in various impacts on certain systems in your body; here's what this looks like:

$$\text{Genetics} + \text{Personality Patterns} \times \text{Loads}$$
$$= \text{Impact on bodily systems}$$

To understand this further, let's explore each of the factors in a little more detail.

Genetics

There is a question I'm asked regularly: 'Is fatigue genetic?' In essence, this means, was my fatigue predetermined by my genes? Was it always going to happen? Well, the level of genetic causation of fatigue in its various forms hasn't been widely studied – just one frustrating example of how fatigue-related conditions have been a casualty of a major lack of funding.

The data we *do* have suggests that there may well be a modest genetic component. For example, one study found that the estimated genetic impact was more than doubled for identical twins (with identical genetics) than with non-identical twins (who are no more related than other siblings). Put another way, if your identical twin has ME/CFS your chance of developing it is twice as high.[74]

Another study, looking at genes in ME/CFS, found 10 relatively common genes, or gene variants, that were significantly more common in people diagnosed with ME/CFS.[75] We could, therefore, easily just assume that fatigue is genetic, and that there is nothing we can do about it. However, if that were the case, there wouldn't be much point in you reading this book, and the OHC approach wouldn't have helped so many people over the years.

So we need to ask ourselves a more fundamentally important question: can our genes be turned 'on' and 'off'? You see, having a genetic predisposition to a disease or a condition only becomes a problem if those genes are activated. As an attempt to answer this question, I think an ongoing study by my friend Dr. Kara Fitzgerald is of particular interest.

Kara and her team were looking at DNA methylation. Without getting too scientific, DNA methylation is a process by which we can change the activity of a DNA segment without changing the sequence.[76] Put another way: they were looking at turning genes on and off!

In the study, participants implemented a series of basic lifestyle changes – including meditation, exercise, and dietary interventions – alongside using specific nutrients known to affect methylation. The finding? After eight weeks, participants who made these changes were measured as being biologically over three years younger. Yes, you read that correctly – eight weeks of lifestyle changes had added over three years to their lives.[76]

The implications of this finding for our health, and specifically our fatigue, is pretty exciting; however, although I think there is some interesting research on its way in the coming years that'll identify the genes that are particularly relevant in fatigue, this will never be the full picture. The way that we live and what happens to us in our lifetimes has a far bigger role to play.

Personality Patterns

Remember our friend Louis Pasteur, the creator of germ theory? Pasteur's entire career was built on the idea that external agents invade our system and make us sick. Well, on his deathbed he purportedly confessed: 'The microbe is nothing, the terrain is everything.'

What Pasteur meant by this is that the presence of the microbe (pathogen) itself is not the defining factor in someone becoming sick – it's more the health of the environment in which the microbe exists. This is why you can expose 10 people to the common cold and perhaps only one individual will catch it. Indeed, every one of us is exposed to countless germs every day but we all know that it's when we're already run-down that we tend to get sick.

What determines the health of the terrain of our body? Well, there are many factors, and we're going to explore them together. But, as we discussed in the last chapter, the state of your nervous system has a direct impact on your mitochondrial function and energy production. And although I'd pretty much fight to the death to defend the argument that fatigue isn't psychological in origin, the way that we live our life has an enormous impact on the health of the terrain of our body.

Indeed, over the years at the OHC we've discovered five key personality patterns that we believe significantly increase the likelihood of developing fatigue. These patterns, which we call 'energy depleting psychologies,' are ways of living our life that are inherently draining and will affect the very terrain in which our cells live. In the next chapter, we're going to explore each of these patterns in detail.

Loads

So, we have our genetic predisposition and we have our personality patterns, but how about the things that happen to us during our lives? Loads represent the many external burdens and events that overload an individual in the years leading up to their becoming fatigued.

As we've touched on, fatigue is almost never caused by one single factor. If a single and acute stress is placed on our system, the chances are that within a relatively short period of time we'll bounce back and recover. If we suffer from ongoing fatigue, it's almost certainly because a series of burdens has been placed on our body over a sustained period of time.

The analogy we use for this is loads on a boat. No one single load on the boat causes it to sink but too many loads, including too many small loads, have a cumulative effect. As the saying goes, 'It's the final straw that breaks the camel's back.'

These loads are any kind of external burden that's placed on us in our lives. Some may stem from childhood, while others may be more recent. Some may have been a one-off, but others may have been ongoing for many years. Furthermore, loads can be psycho-emotional in origin, such as a divorce or financial stress, or physiological, such as exposure to toxic mold or being bitten by a tick and exposed to Lyme disease.

To decode your fatigue, we need to figure out each of those loads and remove them where possible. Ultimately, for healing to happen, we need to create an environment where these burdens on your body are removed. And that's exactly what we'll be exploring in Chapter 7.

Bodily Systems

Your body consists of a number of interlinked systems, each of which has a purpose in its functioning and survival. When these systems aren't working optimally, your health and vitality are immediately affected; examples of bodily systems are your respiratory system, reproductive system, and skeletal system.

Although any of these systems can be impacted by fatigue, our experience is that the nervous system, digestive system, endocrine system, and immune system in particular are affected. Indeed, in

Part II, once we've explored your personality patterns and loads, we'll be looking at how each of these bodily systems is related to your fatigue.

It's also worth noting that multiple bodily systems are usually affected, and they're also impacting each other. For example, if your digestive system isn't working correctly, this may result in hormonal imbalances in your endocrine system, and so perhaps your nervous system will also end up out of balance. Furthermore, they're not discrete systems and they interrelate closely with each other as part of a whole.

Here's a reminder of the formula for map 1, which I hope now makes a little more sense:

Genetics + Personality Patterns × Loads
= Impact on Bodily Systems

Put another way, your genetics and your personality patterns load the gun and the final loads pull the trigger, resulting in the impact on your bodily systems.

Now, this is likely a lot to take in at this point, and please be assured that we'll get into it in a lot more detail in the coming chapters. To bring it alive a little right now, let's revisit the story of Nick the police officer from the last chapter.

Nick may well have had some sort of genetic impact; indeed, this is why he developed chronic fatigue syndrome instead of heart disease, like his colleague. We can then add to this his personality patterns: he was intensely driven by nature; he felt the need to control himself and everything around him; and he was an absolute perfectionist.

On a physiological level, there'd also been a load in the form of a virus, and the series of stressful events at work resulted in a number of significant loads. This all impacted several of Nick's bodily systems, including his digestive, immune, and endocrine systems, and as result, he ultimately developed CFS. In the coming chapters, as we decode your fatigue together, we'll explore how these factors might have come together for you.

Fatigue Map 2: Your Path to Recovery

Now that we've briefly explored map 1, which helps us decode how you became ill, I now want to introduce map 2, the purpose of which is to support your recovery journey. The formula for this map is as follows:

$$\text{State} + \text{Stages} \times \text{Sequence}$$
$$= \text{Healing Impact on Bodily Systems}$$

As before, let's go through each of these factors briefly; we'll look at them in a lot more detail in Part III, as we work together to craft your recovery plan.

State

In order for your body to heal, it has to be in a *healing state*. Even if you weren't in a state of heightened stress and anxiety before you became fatigued, when you're constantly struggling with your energy, your body tends to go into the exact opposite state it needs to be in to heal. And, as we explored in the previous chapter, this has a direct impact on your energy production.

Furthermore, when your energy resources are depleted, the things that were previously not stressful start to become much more so. And you start to live with an ongoing anxiety about how you feel each day – should you rest, should you push through, will you ever feel normal again?

I think an important point to bear in mind is that the body has a powerful and innate capacity for healing. If we cut ourselves, as long as we keep the wound clean and the skin is held together, it will heal. If we break a bone, as long as the bone is set correctly, it won't just mend, the stronger part of the bone will be the location of the break.

In neither of these cases is the source of the injury important – the body has an innate drive and capacity toward healing. When healing doesn't happen, there is a more important question to ask ourselves –

what's stopping us from healing? Well, there are a number of factors, and we're exploring them in this book, but before anything else can be effective, the body has to be in a healing state.

Stages

Have you ever wondered why you can try an intervention at one point in your recovery process and it seems to make your symptoms worse but that same intervention tried at a later stage seems to help significantly? Or vice versa – something that made you feel better earlier now makes you feel worse. This was a phenomenon that caused us significant confusion for many years, until one day I had an epiphany and realized that there are three different *stages* to the recovery process.

Understanding which of these stages we're at is critical for knowing how much activity we should or shouldn't be doing, as well as knowing which interventions are likely to help and which are likely to make things worse. In Chapter 14 we'll get into these three stages of recovery in detail, and we'll use them to help you listen to your body and figure out your activity levels.

Sequence

Understanding the stages of recovery doesn't only help us navigate how much activity we should be doing, it does something equally important: it helps us *sequence* the order in which we use various interventions. You see, different factors are important at different stages. Treatments that might be highly effective at one stage can be seriously harmful at another stage.

As true as the phrase 'One person's medicine is another person's poison' might be, when we start to understand the stages of recovery we also realize that 'One person's medicine at stage 3 of recovery might be the same person's poison at stage 1.'

Sequencing can happen on multiple levels, from the macro of our activity levels and in which order to focus on different therapeutic approaches, to the micro of introducing supplements and dosing.

At this point, the key thing to realize is this: knowing something's good for you isn't enough to tell you *when* it's good for you. Being aware of that alone will be helpful, and we'll come back to this point a number of times within this book.

Bringing it All Together

When it comes to recovering from fatigue, it's critical that we bring each of these ingredients together. Until your body is in a *healing state*, the risk is that nothing else you do is going to be truly effective. We also have to identify which *stage of recovery* you're at, so we know how much activity you should or shouldn't be doing, and we have to work with your body rather than against it for this to be effective.

Once we've established which recovery stage you're at, we need to *sequence* the right interventions in the right order. If we get this wrong, you could be doing exactly the right things at the wrong time and the effect will be negative.

I know this might all sound rather complex, but the purpose of Parts II and III of this book is to help you understand it in more detail and also to map it to your lived experience, so we can work together to decode your fatigue and create your path to recovery.

So, now you've been introduced to the core principles behind the two maps we're going to use to decode your fatigue, it's time to get into them in more detail. Let's start with your personality patterns.

Part II

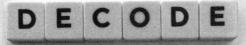

DECODE

YOUR

FATIGUE

Chapter 6

THE PERSONALITY OF FATIGUE

Claire Jones has loved music since she was a little girl. She started out playing the piano and violin but at the age of 10 she heard a musician play the harp and was spellbound. She begged her parents for lessons and, keen to harness such intense passion in one so young, they found her a teacher; three weeks later, she started to learn the harp.

Throughout her teenage years, Claire practiced the harp for hours every day. She gained a place at the Royal College of Music in London, and she performed for anyone and everyone at any opportunity. Playing the harp wasn't just a hobby for Claire – it was her great love.

However, it wasn't until she was 15 that Claire realized what her real dream was. In 2000, Prince Charles, heir apparent to the British throne, restored a position that hadn't been held since 1871 – there would once again be an 'Official Harpist to HRH The Prince of Wales.' The holder of this position would perform on a £150,000 gold-leaf harp made by the famous Italian harp maker Victor Salvi.

In the harp world, there was no greater prize for an aspiring harpist than to play for British royalty. With her heart and mind set on achieving her goal, for the next seven years Claire continued to give everything to the harp. And at the age of 22, she achieved her childhood dream and became Prince Charles's Official Harpist.

For the four years that Claire held the position, she performed for the Royal Family more than 180 times, including at the wedding of Prince William and Kate Middleton. She also released several very successful albums, including *The Girl with the Golden Harp*. Alongside her hectic performing and recording schedule, Claire also took her role as an ambassador for the harp very seriously: she regularly visited schools, helped and guided aspiring harpists, and did all she could to support the next generation of harpists.

To the outside world, Claire had a perfect life. However, the lived reality wasn't quite as it seemed, and her relentless schedule took its toll on her body. Due to being so busy she'd skip meals, she lived in a constant state of stress and anxiety between performances, and there were never enough hours in any given day.

Soon after playing at the Royal Wedding, Claire started to develop debilitating flu-like symptoms and would sometimes need days in bed to recover after performing. In the wake of a particularly demanding tour of the USA, her symptoms became so severe, and she was in so much pain, she could barely climb stairs. And it wasn't just any pain – it was so crippling that no painkiller could touch it.

Claire's symptoms became so concerning that her husband took her to a hospital emergency department, where she promptly collapsed and had a seizure in the corridor. Eventually, she was diagnosed with ME/CFS and was left with a desperately uncertain future, having been told by the conventional medical world that there were no answers.

After several months of being nursed by her mother and husband Chris back in the family home in Wales, and watching as the career she'd given everything to build disappeared in front of her eyes, Claire discovered The Optimum Health Clinic and started working with us via Skype. As is the case for all new patients, an important part of mapping her path to recovery was developing an understanding of how she'd become ill in the first place.

Having been through this process with so many people over the years, we find there are certain tendencies, or personality patterns, that inevitably stand out, and Claire had all of them. However, our discovery of these personality patterns was a journey in itself.

Discovering the Personality of Fatigue

As I reflect on the early years of the OHC, I recall that one of our biggest challenges was the number of patients who appeared to relapse – either on the track to recovery or soon after they'd seemingly recovered. Often, the problem wasn't getting people on the right path, but working out how to keep them on it.

Anna Duschinsky, who founded our psychology department, has worked closely with me over the years to co-develop the Therapeutic Coaching model that's at the heart of our psychology approach. We've had countless long, intense conversations as we've built maps and models around key areas. Having both recovered from ME/CFS ourselves, we also had some rather helpful source material in our lived experience.

One of the things that struck us was that when patients were crippled with severe fatigue, they had little choice but to surrender and rest, at least for a while. Rest was rarely their first choice of strategy – indeed, sometimes it was the last – but with a calmer nervous system, the right nutritional support, and expert input from a practitioner, most people started to make progress.

However, as soon as patients' energy began to return and they had more capacity to live their lives, we noted that their strategy started to change. It was these tendencies and patterns that were of great interest to us. How were people living their lives prior to getting ill, and had that played a role? And what *were* these patterns that were coming back in again as their energy started to return?

The Five Personality Patterns of Fatigue

The model that Anna and I created in those early years has evolved a little since, but much of this has been additional nuance and context on top of the core principles, rather than fundamental changes. We discovered that there are five core personality patterns that are important in fatigue – it's not a definitive list, but in the interests of simplicity, these are by far the most common.

We call these personality patterns 'energy depleting psychologies' because they are ways of approaching ourselves and the world around us that are inherently depleting. You can have one or all of these personality patterns, and different patterns may have different prominence in different chapters of your life.

1: Achiever

Achievers define their self-worth by what they do and achieve in the world. Claire (whose story you've just read) is a classic example of this: from a young age she was driven toward a goal, and everything else in her life became secondary to its obtainment. Oversleeping on the weekend, relaxing with friends, listening to her body when it was tired and needed rest – these all went out the window in the pursuit of her dream.

There were numerous occasions when Claire's body told her it was tired and needed rest; in fact, it was almost like an alarm clock continually going off and trying to get her attention. But she was too busy to listen, and the more drained she became, the more she normalized her body's messages and became numb to them.

The achiever pattern is probably why, in the 1980s, chronic fatigue syndrome was labeled 'yuppie flu.'[77, 78] There seemed to be a disproportionate number of high-pressured executives who were becoming ill. Of course, this pattern is only one small part of a much more complex picture, but the reality still stands – when the body is placed under relentless pressure, at some point it starts to show signs of this.

However, not everyone with an achiever pattern is driven to excel in their career or to gain material status in the world. Indeed, there are many atypical achiever patterns – from being driven to live sustainably and help tackle global issues like climate change, to being the best parent. In truth, there are as many ways to push through the body's feedback in the pursuit of accomplishing things as there are people affected by fatigue.

When I reflect on my own years with chronic fatigue syndrome, I recall that prior to being ill I'd almost rebelled against the pressure that'd been put on me to achieve at school. But when I discovered I could play a direct role in guiding my recovery, it became my playground for achievement, and I gave my entire life to the healing journey. Although one might argue that this was part of the reason why I recovered, I'd make a strong case that if I'd gone a little more gently on myself the journey might have been somewhat shorter.

Whether we're driving ourselves toward our career, trying to make the world a better place, striving to become a good parent, or indeed pursuing our own healing path, if the demands of the tasks ahead of us are consistently placed above our body's communications for rest or care, we're living in a way that's unsustainable, and an achiever pattern is at play.

2: Perfectionist

The perfectionist is a close comrade of the achiever. Perfectionists define their self-worth and create a sense of safety in the world by getting things perfectly right. They tend to have a somewhat black-and-white view of the world, and a sense that there is a right and wrong way of doing things and being on the correct side of this is important.

Perfectionists hold themselves and others to impossibly high standards and often suffer from harsh and unfair internal self-judgment, which they may then also project onto others. Living in the mind and body of a perfectionist can feel utterly exhausting, because however much the body may beg for rest and care, the drive to get things right is more important.

The difference between the achiever and the perfectionist is that the achiever tends to be more focused on the image of success, whereas the perfectionist is more focused on getting things right along the way. Achievers are addicted to the very act of doing and being busy, while perfectionists are addicted to handling all of the details. And of course, we can have both forces at play.

3: Helper

Helpers define their self-worth by what they give to and do for others. They're the classic givers – when it comes to being there for people, nothing is too much trouble for them. This was another personality pattern at play for Claire: on top of the endless demands of her professional role, much of her free time was dedicated to helping and supporting others. If she was asked to run an extra masterclass for aspiring harpists, her response was never 'Do I really have the energy?' but 'How do I fit this into my diary?'

As Anna and I were conceptualizing the helper pattern, she told me stories about the years that she'd been ill. She'd studied for a degree in linguistics at Cambridge University and for much of that period, had battled with dwindling energy. Yet, despite her own deeply challenging situation, she wouldn't think twice about dragging her body out of bed to be there for a friend who was struggling emotionally. It was almost second nature to her – if someone needed support, she'd be there, whatever the cost to her own body.

As with the achiever, there are many different iterations and variations of the helper pattern. For some it may be in the classic sense of being in a helper role, such as a teacher, medic, or therapist. For others, it may be the constant inner pressure to be there for family and friends. And it can be less obvious, too – it may just be the unreasonable demands we place on ourselves to support people in our team at work.

At this point, you may well be thinking, *Hang on, Alex, are you suggesting that to sustain good health we need to live in a world where everyone selfishly looks after their own needs at the expense of everyone else?* No, I'm not. I'm proud to live in a society that values being there for and supporting others, and I also deeply love my job, which allows me to help and care for people.

The issue I'm pointing to is when we constantly ignore our own physical and emotional needs so we can be there for others – not only for an acute period of time, such as supporting a loved one who's going through a crisis, but as a core habit in the way we approach our lives. Ultimately, if we reject and ignore our own needs to be there for others when they need help, we're living our lives in an unsustainable and unhealthy way.

There is a particular challenge that goes with being a helper – because of our natural tendency to want to help others, we find ourselves in a lot of situations with people who want or need our help. Be it full-on codependent relationships or just naturally finding ourselves giving rather than receiving support, the impact is eventually the same – we consistently put more into our relationships than we get back, and this is inherently energy depleting.

This dynamic isn't always the fault of the other person, either – we also teach people how to treat us. Even with those people who aren't naturally energy draining, we'll find that we're the one who's always giving to and taking responsibility for others.

It's also helpful to note that underneath this continual giving to and supporting people we often have a secret hope – if we do enough for others, they'll eventually be there for us and take care of our needs. In a sense, we're giving to others what we hope they'll give to us. The problem with this strategy is that it's utterly flawed. As adults, we're the only ones who can truly know and attend to our needs. That's not to say we can't or shouldn't enlist help or support – we can and should do that – but only *we* can truly be responsible for our happiness.

4: Anxiety

Anxiety types have a constant feeling of being 'on edge' and sense that 'the world isn't a safe place.' There tends to be a lot of mental busyness, and living more in the mind than the body. In essence, the primary strategy is to try and think one's way to a feeling of safety. If we can think of all the possible scenarios around what might happen – how, where, when, why, etc. – and then all of the solutions, we might be able to have a temporary feeling of safety.

It takes a lot of mental energy to fuel this strategy, which means we become less connected to our body and the needs it's trying to communicate to us. This is a fundamentally draining place from which to meet ourselves and the world.

The core problem with anxiety is that it becomes what I call a 'safety loop' (see the diagram below). We feel a feeling of being unsafe in the world, and so our mind speeds up to protect us; as our mind speeds up, we disconnect from our body; by disconnecting from our body we feel more unsafe, and so our mind speeds up further, creating a vicious circle.

Because our nervous system doesn't distinguish between something that's real and something that's vividly imagined, the more anxiety patterns we run, the more draining it becomes to our body and nervous system. In a sense, there is an almost addictive nature to anxiety – we get so used to doing it that we almost can't imagine a world without it.

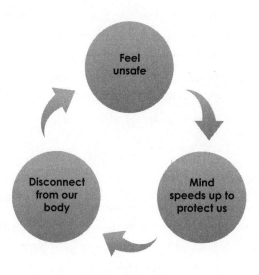

The safety loop

Of course, during a particularly stressful chapter in our life, such as suffering with fatigue, any anxiety patterns we have will become worse. But those with this underlying pattern will be able to trace back their sense that the world isn't quite safe to a time *before* they experienced fatigue.

For some people anxiety is primarily a mental experience, while others will be more aware of the feeling of anxiety in their body. However, when anxiety is felt in the mind it changes what's happening in the body; and equally, when the body is in a state of anxiety it affects the mind.

I should clarify that the anxiety pattern is somewhat different to the maladaptive stress response (MSR), which we'll get to in Chapter 8. The maladaptive stress response is a response to a series of specific stressors, while the anxiety pattern is an underlying strategy for relating to ourselves and the world around us. Whereas MSR is something we can switch off and move on from, if we've a tendency toward anxiety it may be an ongoing thing we're learning to balance in our lives.

For Claire, the busier her schedule became, the more anxiety she started to experience. In a sense, her nervous system was trying to tell her to slow down; however, rather than listen to that feeling, she pushed harder to try and distract herself from her body's feedback loop. This is another common strategy – the worse we feel, the harder we push to try and ignore or change the feeling.

5: Controller

The controller is closely related to the anxiety type. The controller's strategy is to manage the inner sense of not feeling safe in the world by controlling themselves and their environment – be it controlling their emotions, controlling others in a team, or even controlling things such as the temperature in the room or the direction of a conversation.

As with the other personality patterns, sustaining the controller takes an enormous amount of ongoing energy. And because we can't truly control ourselves or the world around us, we're still left with an underlying sense of anxiety. Ultimately, the strategy never truly works.

Furthermore, one of the consequences of the controller pattern is that we tend to push away the people around us who could offer us genuine emotional holding and support. To feel truly supported, we need to be vulnerable enough to let others into our emotional space, and the controller pattern gets in the way of this.

The controller pattern also has a sort of self-perpetuating quality to it – the harder we work to control ourselves and the world around us, the more we generate the illusion that we have some kind of control. This means that the more we do it, the harder it can feel to stop.

Where Do Our Personality Patterns Come From?

It's not uncommon at this point, having had a spotlight shone on each of these personality patterns, to be feeling a little delicate. This is sensitive material, so if there is a critical voice in your mind judging you for having any or all of these patterns, you might want to tell it to go take a hike!

You're also likely wondering whether these patterns are something we're born with or whether they're shaped through our experiences in life. For most people, the answer is both. When I reflect on the origins of my own *achiever* pattern, I can clearly see the conditioning that cultivated it. When I was a child, my mother needed to work multiple jobs to support us financially, so my grandmother played a very active role in parenting my sister and me. Although I believe she was well intentioned, and in her own way very loving, my grandmother placed a heavy emphasis on academic achievement.

I was a relatively bright student and I did quite well at school, but whatever I achieved, it was never enough. If I came second in my class in a test, my grandmother wanted to know who'd come first and why. If I scored 99 out of 100 in an assessment, she was far more interested in the one I'd got wrong than the other 99.

The subtle but clear message was undeniable – love and respect were deeply connected with how much I achieved. If I wasn't up to the mark, love and respect were temporarily withdrawn, and if I excelled, there was the allure that they'd be given. This was only complicated by the fact that the strategy for gaining love and respect in school was the opposite. Indeed, the better I performed in the classroom, the more likely it was that I'd be labeled a nerd or a bookworm. And as one of the most bullied children in the school I attended, this was hardly an appealing prospect.

So, prior to developing CFS, I found myself between a rock and a hard place: achieve at school and be rejected at school, or fail at school and be rejected at home. Regardless of which path I chose, the learning was the same – love is tied to what you do in the world.

When it came to the development of my *helper* pattern, however, that felt rather more innate than conditioned. From a young age, I had an instinctive calling toward helping others. As a young teenager I supported members of my family through the nightmarish events surrounding my sister's mental health issues; and later, when it came to my occupation, it felt like the most natural thing in the world to choose a role in which I could help and support others – it was almost as if it'd always been my destiny.

When you reflect on your own personality patterns, you'll likely notice something similar. Some elements can clearly be mapped to the circumstances of your childhood, while others are just the way that you are. Although understanding the origins of these patterns is both helpful and interesting, it does little to change the fact that they're likely deeply conditioned at this point. To understand how we get free from these patterns, we also need to understand *why* we have them.

The Two Core Needs

These five personality patterns are driven by our attempts to meet two core needs: the need to feel loved and the need to feel safe. For both children and adults, these two needs are at the center of everything – there is almost no limit to what we'll do for love and safety. And if we learn that being loved is linked to what we achieve, what we get right, or how we help others, we'll do everything we can to achieve, perfect, or help. If we learn that our safety in the world is linked to predicting what might go wrong, or controlling ourselves or our environment, we'll give everything we have to do so.

Along the way, Anna and I had a big realization about why so many patients were relapsing – it was because the more energy they reclaimed on the recovery path, the more fuel they had to sustain these personality patterns. When in a crash stage, achievers had to hang up their achieving hats, at least temporarily, and helpers had to restrain themselves from jumping up every time someone was in need. Not because they'd resolved these patterns but because they literally no longer had the energy to sustain them.

Fast-forward a few months into treatment with us and, all things being well, the patient was beginning to see an increase in energy. And what did they start to do with this energy? They got sucked right back into the old personality patterns that'd played a role in their crashing in the first place and found themselves crashing again. With little choice once again, these patterns would be forced back into a temporary hibernation, just long enough for the patient's energy to start to return... and then the cycle would begin again. It was almost as if the body had become allergic to the patient's own personality.

As Anna and I helped people become more aware of their personality patterns, along with working on some of the deeper emotional issues that were fueling them, we noticed that people had smoother recovery paths; and, perhaps more importantly, they learnt ways to live in the world which ensured that their recovery, once it was achieved, would be long lasting.

What Are Your Personality Patterns?

To help create the right foundation for your healing, and avoid potential relapse along the way, we need to take some time to really understand your personality. Indeed, this is the fourth step on our journey together:

Step 4: Understand your personality

As you've been reading the descriptions of the personality patterns in this chapter, I hope there have been some proverbial alarm bells ringing for you. If you want to go deeper into this, I've created a personality rating system as part of the Decode Your Fatigue companion course. It takes about 10 minutes to complete, and I think you'll find it hugely helpful; you can access the course at www.alexhoward.com/fatigue.

The first step in getting free of these patterns is awareness. I've a phrase I often use with patients, 'If you can see it, you don't have to be it.' In other words, the more conscious awareness we have, the easier it is to catch ourselves in the act and *choose* a different path. For example, if we find ourselves about to ignore our own emotional and physical needs because a friend has asked us for support, we can choose to continue down the path toward our self-destruction or instead choose to give ourselves what we really need, deep down.

Cultivating this self-awareness takes practice and discipline. Part of what makes changing our personality patterns challenging is the fact that they're deeply conditioned and there is an unconscious and habitual nature fueling them. It can almost feel like a compulsion that's outside our control. This is because we're not only motivated by our conscious mind but also by our unconscious motivations. By working to calm the influence of these personality patterns, people discover they can neutralize this fuel and find a healthier relationship with their patterns.

When I look at my life now, it's not that I don't have a strong drive toward achieving, or indeed a deep desire to help others and be of service; the difference is that my self-esteem isn't tied to these things. I can challenge myself to achieve things in the world and to be there for others but I'm not doing it in a way that's constantly detrimental to my health and wellbeing.

Cultivating Self-Awareness

One of the tools I use with patients and in my online coaching programs is a 'thought and behavior diary' that helps catch personality patterns as they're happening. The better we get at identifying these behaviors, the easier it becomes to start to change them. It's a simple yet powerful exercise.

1. Every evening, think about the personality patterns we've explored in this chapter, and then write down examples of each one that you've followed that day. These can be big things, such as pushing through your fatigue symptoms all day with an achiever pattern, or subtler ones, such as spending more time than you needed to trying to refine an email with a perfectionist pattern.

2. As you reflect on how these patterns are playing out, that knowledge becomes power. Your next challenge is to get better at catching and stopping those patterns as they're happening.

Let's return to the story of harpist Claire Jones. After 18 months or so of working with the team at the OHC she made a full recovery, and she also discovered a very different way of functioning in the world.

As her own healing journey unfolded, Claire was stunned to discover that many others were suffering in the way she was. She became determined to find a way to help and inspire people in the same situation, and so I invited her to become a patron of our registered charity, which she remains to this day.

I was very grateful to be invited to a recording session for Claire's comeback album, *Journey*. The difference between the Claire who burnt out and the new Claire was dramatic – the same fire and determination were there but she was now taking regular breaks to stretch and move her body. She was also eating properly, practicing meditation and yoga, and managing her schedule in a way that allowed for real balance. Claire realized that changing these patterns wasn't just a temporary shift to get well – it was critical for maintaining her health and maximizing her potential in her career.

Several years later, Claire and her husband Chris welcomed their first child, Cadi, and I was delighted to feature Claire's story in a documentary film we made in 2017. You can watch the film as part of the Decode Your Fatigue companion course; see www.alexhoward.com/fatigue.

Now that we've explored the personality patterns of fatigue, our next step together is to understand the various loads that may have played a role in depleting your system. It's time to make sense of the seemingly unrelated life events that have together gradually impacted your body and impacted your fatigue.

▪▪ Chapter 7 ▪▪

UNDERSTANDING THE
LOADS ON YOUR BODY

D avid was in his late fifties and had just started to enjoy an early retirement after a very successful career as a chief executive in the finance industry. A lifelong music lover, he'd taken up drumming in recent years and with his usual dedication and passion had developed to an impressive standard. For the simple pleasure of playing music, he'd set up his own band and they'd started gigging at local music venues.

David had always enjoyed good health and he'd sustained his wellbeing throughout an intense and demanding career. However, a few years before I met him, he'd been through an immensely challenging time. His wife Leigh had been diagnosed with terminal cancer, and for several long and very painful years he'd been her primary caregiver. Beyond the obvious emotional drain of this, the endless disturbed nights and long hours had also been physically demanding.

Apart from managing his own deep grief at the impending loss of his beloved wife, David was also facing life as a single parent, as well as the need to support his daughter through the unbearable pain of losing her mother. As Leigh's life came close to its end, David was suddenly faced with another huge shock – his father was diagnosed with Parkinson's disease. David was pulled between being there for his wife or for his father, while also supporting his daughter. Eventually, in a period of unimaginable pain, David's wife and father both passed away within a few weeks of each other.

Over the next few years, David did the best he could to keep going and restore a semblance of normal life. He had regular grief counseling, he supported his daughter in every way he could, and he hung on with the precious wish that easier times would come. But they didn't.

Over time, David started to experience a frightening collection of symptoms, among them dizziness, sleep disturbance, and muscle pains. However, his overwhelming symptom was fatigue. This wasn't the kind of fatigue that eases after a good night's sleep or two; instead, it was so crippling that at its worst point he desperately debated whether to ask his daughter to call an ambulance – a course of action he decided against because he doubted he was strong enough to make the journey to hospital.

Despite his dire circumstances, David did have one thing on his side – significant financial resources. And so, over the next few years, he saw countless doctors and medical specialists. Initially, it was thought that he himself might have cancer, and he was forced to face the possibility that his daughter would be left with no one. He had every blood test imaginable and cameras inserted into his body from almost every possible location, and yet the outcome was that no one could explain what was going on.

One night, almost paralyzed by her fear of being alone in the world, David's now teenage daughter was herself desperately searching for answers. She came across the OHC's website and ordered our free information pack. She persuaded her dad to contact us, and I ended up being the person David spoke to. It turned out that David's home was a 10-minute walk from our head office, and so he and I agreed to meet for an initial consultation a few weeks later.

At the OHC, all new patients are asked to complete an in-depth clinical questionnaire; this serves a number of purposes, from helping us screen out potential red flags to giving us important information about someone's case – ultimately, it helps us begin to plan the first steps on their healing journey with us. A key section of the questionnaire asks about certain life events and stressors that patients may have experienced; this includes events from childhood, right up to the present day. As I read David's questionnaire in preparation for our first consultation, it was immediately obvious to me that the events of recent years had played a key role in his becoming ill.

To be clear, I didn't believe that David had fatigue purely because of the loss of his wife and father in such a short period of time. As you're hopefully already learning through our journey together, fatigue is rarely as simple as any one variable. Indeed, underlying vulnerabilities in David's body, his achiever and perfectionist tendencies, and possibly a viral trigger all had their parts to play as well. But if everything else had loaded the gun, his double bereavement had pulled the trigger.

As I explained all this to David during our consultation, I could see him begin to relax in enormous relief. For the first time, his situation made sense, and he also had hope that there might be a path forward. As has been the case for many others like him, I could see a new determination arise in David – he could dare to dream again that things could be different.

Adverse Childhood Experiences

The idea that stressful life events have an impact on our health is certainly not unique to my approach – indeed, it's been a focus of health researchers over the past few decades. A key part of this research was initiated by the US-based insurance company Kaiser Permanente, which provides health services for a fixed fee and as such is highly motivated to maintain and protect the health of its members in order to reduce its long-term liability.

One of Kaiser Permanente's services is a weight-loss program, and in the mid-1980s it was observed that although most participants successfully lost weight on the program, the dropout rate was 50 percent. Vincent Felitti, head of the company's department of preventive medicine, became curious about this and decided to interview some of those who'd quit the program. He discovered that the majority of the 286 people he spoke to had experienced some form of childhood sexual abuse. This suggested to him that weight gain might actually be a coping mechanism for depression, anxiety, and fear.

Felitti teamed up with Robert Anda from the Centers for Disease Control and Prevention (CDC) and they went on to study the childhood trauma experiences of more than 17,000 Kaiser Permanente patient volunteers. In the process of this research, they coined the term 'Adverse Childhood Experiences' or ACEs.

ACEs are defined as 'potentially traumatic events that can have negative, lasting effects on health and wellbeing. These experiences range from physical, emotional, or sexual abuse, to parental divorce or the incarceration of a parent or guardian.'[79]

The findings of the Adverse Childhood Experiences (ACE) study were staggering: the researchers discovered that ACEs were common and that a shocking 28 percent of participants reported physical abuse and 21 percent, sexual abuse. Furthermore, ACEs often occur together – almost 40 percent of those interviewed reported two or more ACEs, and 12.5 percent reported four or more.

The original study has spawned a number of follow-up research papers that have further confirmed and elaborated on these findings. To put this in a real-life context, people who have six or more ACEs have, on average, a 20-year reduction in their lifespan. In recent decades, we've seen a rise in anxiety and stress-related disorders; a rise in insomnia; a rise in diabetes and heart disease. We're flooded with awareness of the fact that our lifestyles are making us ill – the pace and pressure and permanence of it all: utterly unrelenting, wholly unsustainable.

Trauma

Of course, it's not just what happens during childhood that affects our health as adults. Any significant stress or burden in our life will have an effect on our mental, emotional, and physical health. Indeed, David's story is a powerful example of just some of the trauma we can experience in adulthood.

Trauma can happen to us at any age and it isn't just the more obvious things such as physical or sexual abuse or living in a war zone. Trauma is an impact on the mind, emotions, or body that occurs as a result of distressing life events. Put another way, trauma is the result of an overwhelming amount of stress that exceeds one's ability to cope, or to integrate the emotions involved with that experience.

Here are some examples of the trauma we might experience in adult life:

- The death of a loved one

- Divorce

- Moving home

- A major illness or injury

- The loss of a job

And, of course, very often these things happen in sequences. For example, we lose our job and we end up under financial stress; in time, this results in the breakdown of our relationship and we get divorced; the impact of this is that we have to move house, and so on.

As you're reading this, you might be thinking: *Well, Alex, I wasn't sexually abused as a child, and I don't remember being neglected. I also haven't experienced particularly stressful life events, so this doesn't apply to me.* Actually, you're likely wrong.

You see, there are two types of trauma we can experience. There is Trauma with a capital T, which would be the classic trauma described so far. But there is another, much subtler, form of trauma, or what we call trauma with a small 't.' These are developmental traumas that many of us experience; however, just because they're common, it doesn't mean they don't have an impact on our lives. Indeed, ongoing studies suggest it's valid to broaden the scope of ACEs to incorporate less immediate experiences and environments that nevertheless created a sense of ongoing threat.[80, 81]

For example, it might be that while you were growing up, you felt an ongoing sense that the world wasn't a safe place, even though your parents stayed together and your home environment was stable. Perhaps you didn't get the level of physical and emotional holding and reassurance that you needed. Or perhaps you learnt, like I did, that your self-worth and the love of others was deeply entwined with what you did and how much you achieved in the world.

Any childhood that involved your nervous system learning to brace itself against the world, or you having to put your body under unsustainable pressures to be of value in the world, is one that's had some negative impacts on your health as an adult. To be clear, I'm not advocating that children shouldn't be allowed to struggle or that everything should be made easy for them. A childhood in which an individual always gets what they want does little to prepare them for a far from perfect world. However, whether we like it or not, what happens to our physical and emotional body in childhood still affects our health as adults.[82, 83]

Each trauma we experience is another straw on our proverbial camel's back. On its own it may be manageable, but the cumulative effect of too many traumas together must not be underestimated.

The Trauma of Being Ill

There is also another form of trauma – one that it's important to mention at this point. A rarely talked about, and in some cases hugely important, area is the trauma of being diagnosed with, or living with, ongoing fatigue. This is only made worse by the lack of understanding and support from the medical establishment that is experienced by many people suffering from fatigue, as we explored in Chapter 2.

There is some interesting research that shows that the environment we return to after a traumatic incident plays an important role in how negatively it impacts us. For example, soldiers returning from a war zone to a country in which they're respected and valued by society tend to experience less post-traumatic stress disorder (PTSD) than the alternative. It's believed that this is one of the reasons why there was so much PTSD after the Vietnam War: US society wanted to forget the war had happened, and veterans were left to suffer in silence.[84, 85]

If we map this over to fatigue issues, I think there are some similarities. Although I wouldn't for a second wish a serious illness like cancer on anyone, over the years, a number of patients with fatigue issues who were later diagnosed with cancer have told me the latter diagnosis elicited a completely different response from friends and family: those who'd been dismissive and judgmental when these patients had fatigue issues, suddenly became empathic and supportive when they had cancer.

How Trauma Impacts Fatigue

So, what's the actual relationship between trauma, or external life events, and fatigue? Well, for some people fatigue comes out of nowhere – one minute everything seems fine, and the next they're struggling to crawl through each day. For others, there is a gradual weakening of their system over time, sometimes over many years. Indeed, there is a documented association between childhood trauma and developing chronic fatigue syndrome as an adult.

With sudden-onset fatigue medical practitioners can be particularly quick to go looking for the 'trigger' that *caused* someone to get ill. The problem with this approach is that, in my experience, it can be a red herring – it distracts our attention from the many other loads, personality patterns, and genetic signatures that have weakened the system over time and made us vulnerable to that final load.

Furthermore, even if that final load would have been overwhelming for anyone – as in the case of a potent virus and the resulting post-viral fatigue – it still begs the question, why have some people recovered their strength and we haven't?

What Stops People From Healing?

Now at this point you might be thinking, *OK, I've had some stress in my life, but why does the past matter if we can't change it?* Well, there are two reasons why understanding your loads is important:

1. To decode your fatigue, we need to understand the various factors that have caused you to become fatigued in the first place. By identifying the loads on your body throughout your life, we can ensure that healing has taken place where it needs to.

2. If any of these loads on your system are current, they could be a direct block to your recovery journey now.

With regard to the first point, if you have unresolved loads that are still impacting your body, you need to address them. As we'll discuss in the next chapter in a lot more detail, for your body to heal, it has to be in a healing state. And it's very difficult to get in a healing state when your body is still under stress. With regard to the second point, if you have current life stressors that are loading you, it may be that nothing else will be effective until we deal with them.

We don't need to create a *perfect* environment for healing to happen; however, we do need to create a situation where your body is able to consistently build more energy than it's spending. Indeed, this brings us to the fifth of our 12 steps together:

Step 5: Create an environment for healing

For some of us, creating the necessary environment for healing isn't an easy thing. It can mean leaving a toxic relationship, or walking away from a demanding career that we feel defines our value in the world. It can also mean prioritizing our own rest and healing over the many things we've got used to doing for others. However, in some cases, until these changes take place, healing simply cannot happen. For healing to happen, we have to create an environment within which it's possible.

What Are Your Loads?

Let's now do some homework together. I want you to take a little time to identify the major stressors you've experienced in your life. From your childhood right up to the present day, what are the major life events that have caused stress for your body, and indeed may still be doing so now? These could be:

- Divorce or the end of a relationship

- Financial stress or the loss of a job

- Stressful circumstances at work

- Loss of a loved one

- Physical injury or major surgery

- Physical or sexual abuse

- Being abandoned as a child by a parent

- Lack of emotional nourishment and holding as a child

Do you feel that any of these events are still impacting you today? Are they getting in the way of your body being able to heal? What do you need to do to cultivate the ultimate environment for healing today?

Let's return to David's story. In the year following his first consultation with us, David went through the very program you're learning in this book, and I'm pleased to say he later made a full recovery. Indeed, once on the other side he reported feeling the best he'd felt in his life, despite then being in his early sixties.

I'm also pleased to say that David's story didn't end there. He fell in love once again and remarried a few years later. And, determined to give something back to the approach that had transformed his life, he asked if there might be a way to use his many years of organizational experience to help support us. In time, he became a trustee of our registered charity, and then chairman, as well as an important mentor for me.

David also decided that he missed the challenges of his working life, and he returned to a full-time and very fulfilling career as a non-executive director in multiple roles in financial services. He and I remain good friends to this day. You can watch the documentary film of David's story on the Decode Your Fatigue companion course at www.alexhoward.com/fatigue.

We've explored the impact of your personality patterns, and the various loads of your life, and so now it's time to take a fascinating dive into the state of your nervous system, and discover whether or not your body is wired for healing.

■■ Chapter 8 ■■

ARE YOU IN A HEALING STATE?

Colin was in his early thirties and was used to living a full and dynamic life. By day he worked for a tech company in London and by night he ran a recording studio with friends, producing music – they'd even had modest success in the dance-music charts.

When Colin started to show signs of burnout, it came as no real surprise to him or anyone else; he'd been burning the candle at both ends for years. His achiever personality pattern was obvious, even to those who weren't aware of such a thing.

At the time, I'd been practicing as a therapist for just over a year, and Colin was one of the first clients I worked with who was suffering from ME/CFS. A friend of a mutual friend had recommended my first book to him, and he was hopeful that I could help. The person who'd put us in touch was training as a nutritional therapist and was working with Colin on that level, and so he was looking for my help on the psychology side.

The Optimum Health Clinic was still only a few months old and based in a modest room in the house where I lived in North London. There was a bed in one corner, a kitchen in another corner, and a large desk taking up the rest of the room; thankfully, there was a rather nicer room in the basement, which I rented by the hour to see patients.

Colin and I sat down together in the comfortable leather chairs and he told me about his background. He explained that he'd recently been diagnosed with ME/CFS after suffering with debilitating symptoms for the previous six months. He'd been forced to stop work and was now feeling deeply frustrated and desperate for answers.

The frenetic and insatiable pace with which Colin asked questions was a telltale sign that he had a strong predisposition toward anxiety. It was clear to me that this was certainly not helping his body to heal, and it would be a good place to start. Over the next hour I taught Colin several techniques that would help calm and settle his nervous system, and we then made an appointment to meet again in a few weeks.

A week later, I received an email from Colin. He'd found our session helpful, he told me, and what I'd said had made a lot of sense to him; however, he was having a crash and his symptoms were as bad as ever. Was there anything he could do before our next session to help ease things?

I suggested that we have a phone call later that day to chat things through. Colin's frustration at his symptoms, and his anxiety about what was happening, were palpable. Every response I gave to a question triggered three more questions. I didn't have such clarity at the time, but what Colin was trying to do was think his way to a feeling of safety that would allow him to relax somehow.

However, as we touched on in the last chapter, such a strategy makes things worse rather than better. It was clear to me that Colin was in exactly the opposite state to the one he needed to be in to heal, and before anything could have a chance of working, we needed to calm down his system.

Within the school of Neuro-Linguistic Programming (NLP) there is a technique called the 'As if frame,' which works as a sort of thought experiment – you act 'as if' something is true, even though you know it might not be. For example, you might act *as if* everything in your life has happened for a positive reason, or *as if* everything in a particular situation is going to turn out as you hope.

I had an idea for using this tool with Colin: I suggested we act 'as if' his entire physical state was a direct result of his mental and emotional state. Therefore, if he committed absolutely to calming his nervous system over the coming week, perhaps that would have a direct impact on his symptoms. Doing so meant that he wouldn't check his symptoms and worry about them; that he wouldn't keep researching his condition in a panicked bid to find answers; and that he wouldn't restrict everything in his life on the basis of his illness – although he would continue to respect his symptoms and listen to his body.

Put another way, we were going to pretend that Colin was well and the only thing he needed to do was stop thinking about his symptoms – and stop his mind when it started to do so; for this, he'd use several tools that would break and retrain his thought patterns. Somewhat tentatively, Colin agreed to the experiment and I taught him the tools; if nothing else he was excited to have something to play with over the coming week. After the call, I didn't think much more about this conversation and went back to my day's work.

The following week, as I heard Colin arrive for his session, I remembered what we'd discussed on the phone and wondered how he was doing. As I opened the door to greet him I saw that he was like a different person – his face was lighter, his eyes were brighter, he looked about five years younger, and he had a spring in his step.

Colin went on to tell me about what he could only describe as a miracle. Not only had he bounced back from his crash, his energy had also shot up, he'd been out seeing friends, and he'd even spent an evening at his recording studio with no ill effects; and for the first time in a long while he was enjoying life. He couldn't *believe* what'd happened. And the truth was, neither could I. I knew the techniques I worked with were effective, but this was a stunning confirmation for me of just how powerful the mind can be.

Does this mean that Colin's illness was in his mind and all he needed to do was stop thinking about it? Absolutely not – in fact, Colin's full recovery took several more years from that point and the use of many of the other principles we're going to come to in this book. But it was a huge turning point in his healing path, and it was also a big turning point in my professional career.

What Is Stress?

Stress is a word that's thrown around a lot these days. It tends to conjure up images of executives rushing around with a mobile phone attached to each ear, but stress is so much more than that.

Stress was once seen as a sign of weakness, but these days it's almost a badge of honor for someone who's hustling hard in their life. It's a common belief that if we're not stressed, then we're not pulling our weight and working hard. To fully understand the concept of stress, I think we need to clarify what it actually is.

Before the famous Austrian endocrinologist Hans Selye did his groundbreaking research on the effects of stress on the human body, the term 'stress' was used in physics to describe physical force on an object that exceeds its ability to meet that force. From this perspective, stress is ultimately when the demand placed on something exceeds the supply of resource to meet it.

The Three Types of Stress

Of course, in human beings stress is more complex than that. Two people can be presented with the same external stress and have a different response to it. To help us make sense of this, my friend Dr. Heidi Hanna talks about three different types of stress:

1. **Stress load**: as outlined in the physics definition above, this relates to the stress load we're placed under.

2. **Stress lens**: this term refers to how we perceive the stress placed in front of us. For example, two people are presented with a roller coaster, and while one looks at it through the lens of excitement and adventure, the other sees it through the lens of fear and terror.

3. **Stress signature**: each person's nervous systems is wired slightly differently and, as we'll discuss in Chapter 10, if we have weak adrenal glands, we may find that when it comes to handling stress, our resilience is less than that of someone who doesn't. Or, if we've experienced trauma in previous relationships, we might notice a particular sensitivity to rejection and have a greater stress response when others ignore us.

Therefore, for us as individuals, our stress is defined as the *stress load* we face, the perspective *or lens* through which we perceive that load, and the *physical resources* we have to deal with it.

Understanding the Stress Response

To understand how stress affects our body, we have to understand its biological origins. What's known as our 'stress response' goes right back to our caveman days... Let's say you and I are sat around the campfire together, toasting some tasty pieces of buffalo and sharing stories about the day's adventures. Suddenly, out of the corner of your eye, you spot a saber-toothed tiger prowling in the bushes, and the look on its face says it's not eaten a decent meal for a few days.

In that moment you're going to get an enormous hit of the stress hormones adrenaline and cortisol, and we both have three choices available to us: fight, flight, or freeze. Let's explore each of these in detail.

Fight

If we're armed with some kind of spear, and we're feeling up to the challenge, we could take on the saber-toothed tiger in a fight to the death. If you're game, go for it, but it's not my preferred choice!

Flight

We can attempt to escape. Perhaps we can climb a tree, or maybe we fancy ourselves as distant ancestors of Usain Bolt and believe we can outrun our furry friend. I'm not a fast runner, but this one gets my vote!

Freeze

On the off chance that the saber-toothed tiger hasn't yet seen us, we may choose to stay very still and hope that it doesn't. Or, if it has seen us, we also have the option of playing dead and pretending we're not a threat (I'm not keen on this choice because in this instance, our friend is looking rather hungry.)

Whichever of these responses you and I choose, our biology will undergo a somewhat miraculous and fairly instantaneous transformation under the direction of our autonomic nervous system.[86] Our nervous system has two primary modes: the job of our sympathetic nervous system is to prepare us for action, while the job of our parasympathetic nervous system is to calm this response and allow our system to 'rest and digest.'

In the sympathetic nervous system response, the blood flow to our skeletal muscles and lungs is enhanced by as much as 1,200 percent. Our body starts pumping with hormones such as adrenaline and cortisol, which give us temporary superhuman abilities.

At the same time, blood flow is directed away from functions such as digestion – which is why when we're under stress we can suffer from constipation or diarrhea. After all, if we're about to be eaten by a saber-toothed tiger, digesting our buffalo dinner is no longer a biological priority.

Now, let's assume that we're lucky enough to survive our encounter with the saber-toothed tiger – after all, if we don't, it's all a bit of a moot point anyway. Once we know that we're safe, we don't need that massive hit of stress hormones and our muscles and lungs can return to normal levels of blood flow. It's now time to go back to digesting whatever is left of the buffalo in our digestive system – i.e. our parasympathetic nervous system kicks in.

To keep things simple, I refer to these two fundamental states as a stress state and a healing state. A stress state is the product of the sympathetic nervous system's fight-or-flight response (or an extreme parasympathetic nervous system shutdown or freeze state) while a healing state is a parasympathetic calming response. The process of transitioning between these two states is at the core of our biology, and we have it to thank for our survival over the millennia.[87, 88]

Indeed, a state of stress isn't just a necessary function for our survival – we also grow and adapt when under stress.[89] For example, when we go to the gym and lift weights, we're deliberately stressing our muscles so they grow. Stress isn't inherently bad, but it becomes a problem when our stress response becomes maladaptive. A maladaptive stress response is when our stress response gets stuck on 'on' even when it doesn't need to be. Ultimately, things that shouldn't be stressful become so, and our nervous system is in the exact opposite state to what it needs to be in to heal (more on this in a moment).

Acute Stress vs. Chronic Stress

The type of stress we experienced thousands of years ago in our caveman days was typically sudden and immediate stress: there was a threat in the environment and we either survived it or we didn't. This is the kind of acute stress that our body has evolved to deal with.

The kind of stress we experience in the modern world is often very different. Yes, we might experience an acute, sudden stress, such as when we step off the curb into the road and are almost knocked down by the enormous lorry we failed to spot; however, such forms of stress are the exception rather than the rule.

Consider a typical day... We're jolted awake by an alarm clock and then rush around the house getting ready for work. Before leaving, we pump our body full of caffeine to wake us up, and then fight our way through traffic (literally risking life and limb).

At work, we deal with information and demands coming from every direction, and throughout the day we continue using caffeine, sugar, and other stimulants to keep our tired system awake. The frenetic pace doesn't end when we get home. In the evening, we're still connected to the world through email and social media, right up until the minute we go to sleep. In the modern world it's as if the saber-toothed tiger is chomping at our backside all day long. And, unlike our ancestors, we tend not to discharge the stress we're holding in our body with regular physical activity.

Are You Living Like a Frog?

With all this talk of stress, you might now be thinking, *Alex, that's all well and good – and I can see what you're saying in other people – but I don't feel stressed.* Here's the thing: human beings have an amazing ability to normalize and adapt to their environment. It's another part of our evolved ability to survive almost any environment.

It's not an experiment I've done, or one that I'm recommending, but I'm told that if you drop a frog into a bowl of boiling water it'll leap right out. Its fight-or-flight response kicks in and literally saves its life.

However, if you take that same frog, put it into a bowl of cold water and slowly heat the water, it'll stay in the bowl and boil to death. Why? Because it keeps normalizing to the increase in the water's temperature.

The same thing happens to human beings – we're biologically programmed to adapt to whatever environment we're in. I've had patients who are so flooded with stress hormones they're unable even to sit still in their chair and tell me that they're *not* stressed. I feel stressed just sitting across from these people, but for them it's just a normal, everyday experience.

The Lens of Fatigue

What does all this mean in the context of fatigue, particularly severe fatigue? Perhaps you're thinking, *How can I possibly be stressed? I barely leave the house. My life used to be stressful, but feeling stressed now would almost feel like progress.* But here's the thing: suffering from a medically unexplained illness is in itself a deeply stressful experience.

With a more predictable illness, however difficult or challenging it might be, the diagnosis and prognosis do at least give us clarity. The unpredictable and fluctuating nature of fatigue gives us anything but the certainty we crave. When we don't know *what's* wrong with us, *why* it's wrong with us, and *whether* we'll even recover, it's immensely stressful to our system. Our mind can end up incessantly asking questions: should we rest, should we push through, are we going crazy, or do people think it's all in our mind?

Indeed, in an attempt to keep us safe, our mind goes into an almost obsessive pattern of checking symptoms, attempting to make sense of them, and trying to decide whether we should do something or not. As this pattern evolves, even the simplest things can become an enormous source of stress. Our entire world becomes viewed through the lens of our fatigue.

Put in the language of Dr. Heidi Hanna, we might already be struggling with our stress load, and our stress signature is likely also an issue, but our stress lens then also becomes distorted. In our constant attempts to keep ourselves safe from our frightening symptoms, we develop a mental program through which the entire world is filtered. Many adults are pre-programmed as children, through the adverse childhood experiences we discussed earlier, to be prone to this type of response.[82]

If you think about a computer operating system, it's the program through which all other programs are run. For example, if your computer is a Mac, you'll be running a version of the OS X operating system, whereas if you're on a PC, you'll be running a version of the Windows operating system. In the early years of the clinic, some of our computers were running on Windows Millennium Edition, otherwise known as Windows ME. We had all kinds of problems with this software – it didn't seem to be able to run multiple programs together and it kept crashing – so we gave the mental program I've just described the name 'Windows ME.'

You see, like a computer, the brain has certain central programs through which everything else is computed and processed. Consider for example someone who holds the belief that all people are bad and are out to get us. From a harmless glance from a stranger in the street to their own intimate and family relationships, they'll have a very different way of making sense and meaning of the world than someone who believes that people are inherently good and kind.

When we're suffering from fatigue, there is an enormous amount of uncertainty from day to day – doing too much activity can have merciless consequences and our symptoms can be genuinely frightening, which is only compounded by the experts' inability to explain to us why we have them.

Think back to Colin, whose story started this chapter. After a number of months of worsening symptoms that were mysterious and scary in nature, Colin was becoming obsessed with and terrified of his fatigue. The first thing he did when he woke up in the morning was scan his body for symptoms, and this would continue throughout the day. Something as simple as an invitation to a dinner party would trigger thoughts like, *Will I have the energy? Will I crash afterward?* As Colin's fatigue increased when he did any kind of activity, his stress response got worse and worse, to the point where it became paralyzing.

And, in case you're wondering if anxiety about our symptoms can really have that much impact, remember that the body doesn't distinguish between something that's real and something that's vividly imagined. This is why someone with a spider phobia can literally pass out through fear at even the suggestion there might be a spider in the room. It's not the spider that causes them to pass out – it's the *idea* of the spider. It's the same mechanism that occurs when we imagine eating our favorite meal and our mouth begins to salivate.

The Maladaptive Stress Response

I hope that after our tour through the physical elements of fatigue you realize that I'm not for a second suggesting that the symptoms of fatigue aren't real – nothing could be further from the truth. And yet, when we're living with a medically unexplained illness that involves frightening and confusing symptoms that are fluctuating in nature, it has an impact on our nervous system. As a result of living with these symptoms, our sympathetic nervous system becomes chronically activated and we end up in a stress state rather than its opposite – a healing state.

In itself, stress isn't a problem, and neither is our body's response to stress. But with fatigue, this stress response often becomes maladaptive because we end up stuck in a state of chronic stress. For many people, addressing this maladaptive stress response is a critical part of the healing journey.[90–92]

And, if you think back to Chapter 4, beyond everything else we've talked about in this chapter, a maladaptive stress response directly impacts our mitochondria, which are the energy powerhouses of our cells. When we're in a maladaptive stress response, our body creates less energy.

This brings us to our next step. For our body to heal, we have to be in a healing state:

Step 6: Get in a healing state

Calming the nervous system is a significant piece of work. Indeed, it's the core focus of my online coaching program, the RESET program, during which, over a 12-week period, I teach and support people in using a powerful set of techniques and practices to rewire their system. In Chapter 15 we'll get into some of the basics of this program together, but for the purposes of this chapter, I first want to build your awareness of the current state of your nervous system with the following exercise.

Are You In a Stress State or a Healing State?

Your body can be in one of two states – a stress state or a healing state. For your body to heal, it needs to be in a healing state. The first step to calming your nervous system is identifying which state you're in. Consider the following questions:

1. Do you find yourself feeling tired and wired?

2. Do you struggle to switch off and sleep at night?

3. Do you find yourself checking and thinking about your symptoms a lot of the time?

4. Does your mind race?

5. Do you find it hard to relax your body fully?

6. Are you reactive to many supplements, foods, chemicals, and so on?

If you've answered yes to some of these questions, it's likely that your body is in a maladaptive stress response at least some of the time.

It's very easy to gloss over the importance of what we've explored together in this chapter, but until the body is in a healing state, my experience is that little else will work. Indeed, this is also an example of why our dual approach of functional medicine and psychology is so critical at the OHC. When people get stuck and can't move forward on the physical side, very often a shift in their nervous system on the psychology side will be the key to unlocking things.

Now, at this point I'm mindful that I may appear to have overemphasized the importance of psychology. That hasn't been my intention, although experience has shown me that these pieces need to be in place before we move forward – in fact, we ignore these at our peril on the healing journey. In the next chapter, we're going to take a fascinating dive into the world of the digestive system and explore the exact process the body uses to break down food into the raw ingredients your mitochondria need to make energy.

■■ Chapter 9 ■■

YOUR DIGESTIVE SYSTEM – BREAKING DOWN YOUR ENERGY SOURCE

Some years before I crashed with chronic fatigue and my life fell apart, I started to experience crippling digestive symptoms. These would come and go, but at times I'd be in agonizing pain that could only be relieved by a very large and very uncomfortable bowel movement. At the time I called them 'stomach pains' because I didn't really understand that our digestive system is so much more than just our stomach.

Following several visits to our local doctor, I was sent to see a gastroenterologist. After going through some rather invasive and uncomfortable tests, I was told they could find nothing wrong with me, and I was given the diagnosis of irritable bowel syndrome (IBS). I remember at the time thinking that this was hardly a diagnosis – just as I would later with my chronic fatigue syndrome diagnosis – my symptoms were simply repeated back to me with the word 'syndrome' on the end.

I was sent away with some pills to take when I had a flare up of IBS, but these turned out to do nothing whatsoever. As far as I can recall, not once during this process of investigation and diagnosis was I asked what I ate. When you think about it, that's pretty crazy – if a car's engine kept breaking down for no apparent reason, one of the first things you'd check was the fuel that's being put into it.

If someone had bothered to ask, they'd have discovered that my diet featured enormous quantities of sugar, fizzy drinks, and chocolate. My family *did* try to feed me healthy food, but I had a sweet tooth and I was stubborn. This meant that at school I'd often throw away my healthy packed lunch and replace it with a chocolate bar or two.

When I developed chronic fatigue a few years later, one of the first practitioners I saw was the pioneering environmental doctor John Mansfield. He *did* ask me what I was eating, and he also looked into my body's ability to digest it. A quarter of a century later, some of Dr. Mansfield's interventions do seem rather outdated; however, that in itself is a testament to how far things have evolved because of the extraordinary foundations that he and several others established.

You Are What You Absorb

Take a step back in your mind to Chapter 3, when we talked about your mitochondria, the powerhouses of cellular energy production. What was the first step in the cycle? That's right, the food we eat. In fact, it was Hippocrates, the founding father of modern medicine, who, around 460–370 BCE, said that 'All disease begins in the gut.'

We all know the phrase 'You are what you eat,' but in fact, this is only part of the story. You're not just what you eat, you're what you *absorb*, and when it comes to decoding your fatigue, your ability to digest and absorb food is critical. If your digestive system isn't working effectively, your mitochondria won't get the ingredients they need to make energy, and everything else will go out of balance.

Your Amazing Digestive System

Your digestive system, also known as the gastrointestinal tract or the gut, is rather more than just your stomach, and it's pretty incredible. Did you know that...

- The gastrointestinal tract is approximately 32 ft (9.5 m) long and its surface area is 322–430 ft² (30–40 m²), which is around the size of a small apartment.

- It's through your gastrointestinal tract that the outside world contacts your inside world, which is why 70–80 percent of your immune system is found there. The structures and functions along your gastrointestinal tract have evolved to allow the right things to be brought in (nutrients, water) and the wrong things (everything else) to be kept out.

- The gastrointestinal tract is home to an entire ecosystem – trillions of microorganisms known collectively as the gut microbiome.[93] This population of bacteria, viruses, fungi, yeasts, and other organisms plays a crucial role in maintaining your health and wellbeing. Indeed, in the human body, microbial cells outnumber human cells by a factor of 10.[94]

The Gut–Brain Axis

A key element in understanding why your digestion impacts your fatigue – as well as symptoms such as brain fog and cognitive function – is being aware of the relationship between the microbiota in your gastrointestinal tract and your brain. Research has shown there is two-way communication between the brain and the gut microbiome via the central nervous system – this is known as the gut–brain axis. Indeed, in recent years scientists have started to refer to the gut as 'the second brain.'

One of the key functions of your gut microbiome is safeguarding the integrity of the barrier that is your gut wall. Your microbiome can be negatively impacted by a number of factors, including poor dietary choices, stress, and long-term use of some medications.

Research suggests that imbalances in the gut microbiome may be associated with changes in memory, anxiety, mood, and stress response, and can directly impact the integrity of the blood–brain barrier that safeguards the brain.[95–97, 98–102] Ultimately, issues with your gut directly influence, and sometimes cause, symptoms such as brain fog, joint pain, and eczema.[103]

A Journey Through the Digestive Process

Indeed, your digestion is so important for healing your fatigue that it's the next step in our 12-step plan:

Step 7: Optimize your digestion

To optimize your digestive function, we need to take a methodical approach to the various imbalances that can arise. The journey taken by your food – from your plate to providing energy in your cells – is a complex one, and the nutrients it contains can encounter many roadblocks en route. A simple way to think about it is that your digestive system, or gastrointestinal tract, is a series of connected sections, each with a different function, that form a long, twisting tube from your mouth to your anus (see diagram below), and at each stage along the way, a multitude of things can go wrong.

The easiest way to decode your digestion is to take a journey through the digestive process; in this way, you'll see what happens at each stage, understand what can go wrong, and explore what we can do to offer support.

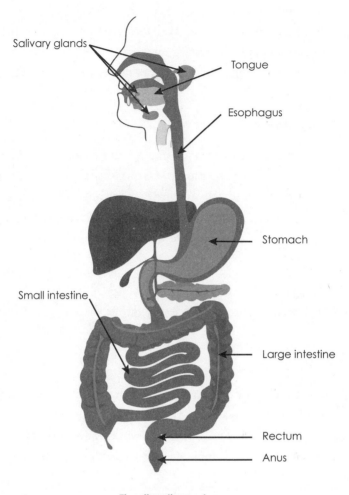

The digestive system

Stage 1: The Mouth

Before we even put food in our mouth, the digestive process has started. The sight, smell, and even thought of food triggers the production of saliva in our salivary glands, which contains special enzymes to help initiate the digestive process.

Once food enters our mouth, we have the critical job of chewing it, which effectively increases the available surface area of the food, allowing better access for digestive enzymes. The better we chew our food, the easier it is to digest and the more nutrients we can take from it.

What Can Go Wrong?

When we eat mindlessly, without paying attention to our food – for example, eating while on the move, in front of the television, or during meetings – we tend not to chew properly. This means we're swallowing partially chewed food, which from the outset leaves the rest of our digestive system with more work to do.

And if we eat in a state of stress, it can have an influence on our whole digestive function, as our body is in a state of sympathetic nervous system dominance (fight, flight, freeze) rather than 'rest and repair.'[104]

How We Address It

It might sound rather simplistic, but ensuring you chew each mouthful of food 20 times before swallowing it, eating meals in a quiet place where you can be in tune with your body, and working to calm your nervous system before eating (we'll look at ways to do that in Chapter 15) can have a significant impact.

Stage 2: The Stomach

Your stomach has a capacity of around 1 quart (1.5 liters). Every day, it produces around 4 pints (2 liters) of gastric juice, which plays a key role in breaking down food, and also in your immune response – by killing bacteria or germs that might try to enter your body. The cells of your stomach produce a combination of hydrochloric acid, mucus, and digestive enzymes; these all facilitate the breakdown of food into a combined, soup-like mix called chyme.

What Can Go Wrong?

There are a number of conditions that occur in the stomach that should be reviewed by a medical professional, including hiatus hernia, gastric ulcers, gastritis, Helicobacter pylori (H. pylori) infection, stomach cancer, and pernicious anemia.

From our perspective, two of the key considerations at this point in the digestive process are the effective production of hydrochloric acid and digestive enzymes. If our production of these crucial elements is suboptimal, undigested food may pass into the small intestine. Even a perfect diet isn't perfect unless we can break foods down into nutrients small enough to be absorbed further on in the gastrointestinal tract.

How We Address It

If there are indications that something might be going wrong at this stage, it's important to get appropriate medical input to rule out other causes, such as those outlined above. It's also important to explore levels of hydrochloric acid and digestive enzyme. If these are found to be deficient, this can be addressed by the use of supplements, which can lead to significant improvement.

It's also important to avoid overfilling the stomach. When we eat too much food in one go, even normal levels of hydrochloric acid and digestive enzymes won't be enough to break the food down, and we'll again end up with undigested food.

Stage 3: The Small Intestine

The small intestine is a tube that's around 23 ft (7 m) long and has random twists and turns. At the top of this section of the gut, where it joins the stomach, the gallbladder and pancreas release further enzymes to aid with digestion. There is a high concentration of immune cells in your small intestine and if your immunity is overactive here you may experience food intolerances; if it's underactive, you may be prone to general infections.

The majority of our nutrient absorption takes place in the small intestine, via the tiny fingerlike structures called villi that project inward from its lining. There are around 30 villi per square mm, each of which are covered by microvilli to maximize the surface area available for nutrient absorption. It's through your small intestine villi that food is absorbed into your body.

Every four hours, the 'migrating motor complex' sweeps the small intestine – it's kind of like this organ's cleaning process. You'll feel it as that gurgling/rumbly tummy sensation, and it's a sign that things are working well.

What Can Go Wrong?

One of the most common digestive issues in fatigue patients is known as increased intestinal permeability, or more commonly, 'leaky gut.'[105, 106] This is simply an indication that the integrity of the gut is compromised because the so-called tight junctions that make up the gut wall are less secure than they should be.

In a leaky gut the usually carefully policed system that allows only specific molecules into the body instead permits the increased entry of elements such as undigested food particles, pathogens, and toxins. When the immune system sees something in the blood it doesn't recognize, it activates an immune response, which may lead to inflammation.

The greater the level of increased intestinal permeability, and the greater the entry of 'unchecked' elements into the body, the greater the potential for immune activation, inflammation, and food and chemical sensitivities. This in turn triggers a vicious cycle – the more inflammation and immune activation there is in the body, the greater the risk of damage to the gut wall (resulting in poor nutrient absorption), and the greater the pressure on mitochondrial health and energy production.

So how do we end up with a leaky gut? Well, there are many books on this subject alone, but the most common cause is an imbalance in the gut microbiome (the ecosystem of bacteria that live within us), otherwise known as gut dysbiosis.[107] For many years the blame for dysbiosis was laid almost exclusively at the door of candida, a yeast that can cause fungal overgrowth. I was one of many people who went on aggressive anti-candida programs and I believe there was some long-term damage to my gut microbiome as a result.

These days, there is a lot more research on and interest in gut health. The latest surge has been around small intestinal bacterial overgrowth (SIBO); this is where there is an overgrowth of potential 'good' and 'bad' bacteria in the small intestine, which, compared to the large intestine, is supposed to be a relatively sterile environment.[108–111]

How We Address It

Addressing fungal overgrowths such as candida, bacterial misplacement such as SIBO, and general dysbiosis or microbiome imbalances effectively and safely requires the input of an experienced practitioner. There are various antimicrobial protocols that can be very effective, and for SIBO there are very specific antibiotics that are well tolerated (and are not absorbed beyond the gut, meaning they're much less likely to have unnecessary systemic effects).

In recent years there has been a paradigm shift that really emphasizes the importance of supporting a healthy balance of microbes in the gut microbiome, rather than just focusing on the eradication of 'bad bacteria.' This support pays attention to the fact that fostering a favorable environment in the gut – with the right elements to encourage the growth of good bacteria and mucus membranes – is key.

It's also worth bearing in mind that encouraging bacterial diversity in the gut is essential, and generally much more effective than harsh microbial eradication approaches. This is why an experienced practitioner is key to ensuring that the approach chosen is balanced and considers all elements of your individual gastrointestinal profile; this can include using different forms of probiotics.

Diet is also very important in addressing gut dysbiosis. We'll explore some food fundamentals in Chapter 16, but of particular importance is avoiding sugar and too many carbohydrates, which will feed bad bacteria.

For some fatigue sufferers, avoiding refined carbohydrates can be critical. One particularly common example of this is the FODMAP group of foods (which stands for Fermentable Oligosaccharides, Disaccharides, Monosaccharides and Polyols); FODMAPs occur in a wide range of foods, from apricots and apples to cows' and goats' milk, and cashew nuts and chickpeas, and for some people they can be a consistent trigger of food intolerance reactions.

Stage 4: The Large Intestine

The large intestine is a quarter of the size of the small intestine, at 5 ft (1.5 m) in length, and includes the colon, rectum, and anus. Food arrives in the large intestine around eight hours after it's eaten, and an entire meal can take up to a week to be entirely eliminated. We should have an average of 1–2 bowel movements a day, and stools should be formed (not runny, but not hard).

Among the other functions in the large intestine, water is absorbed and feces are formed. Our large intestine also houses the majority of our gut microbiome; this community of microorganisms assists in further digestion of carbohydrates, turning them into fuel for the cells of the gut wall, and to be used elsewhere in the body. The microbiome has a plethora of other duties to perform, including producing some vitamins, protecting the gut wall, contributing to the workings of the gut–brain axis – including influencing our moods – and supporting a healthy immune system.

What Can Go Wrong?

A number of medical conditions can occur in your large intestine – among them are inflammatory bowel disease (IBD), diverticulosis, appendicitis, bowel tumors, and Crohn's disease (which can attack any part of the digestive tract). As with the small intestine, there can also be issues with dysbiosis, such as candida.

Furthermore, in the large intestine we can experience issues with parasites. These organisms effectively feed on us as a host and can produce localized symptoms as well as more systemic ones such as fatigue, fever, and flu-like symptoms.

Of particular relevance in the large intestine is the frequency of our bowel movements – from constipation, when our bowel movements are too infrequent, to extreme diarrhea, when we're having too many and stools may be poorly formed.

How We Address It

Many of the principles for working with the small intestine also apply to the large intestine, along with the need for tailored protocols for things such as parasites – this might involve antimicrobials to kill parasites, and ensuring we control our exposure to further infection, be that via pets, hand/mouth transmission, unwashed foods, etc.

And remember, it's critical to populate and encourage the development of a healthy microbiome. A powerful tool for this can be taking probiotics, which essentially feed our gut with 'good' bacteria.

If there are issues with the volume and frequency of bowel movements, understanding what's causing this and addressing it is also important.

Adding fiber-rich foods to our diet, ensuring we're sufficiently hydrated, and addressing food intolerances can also be important.

Next Steps

In Chapter 16 we're going to get into food and what you should be eating, but when it comes to addressing the various things that can go wrong with our digestive function, often we'll need to work with a nutritionist trained in functional medicine. They'll gather a full clinical picture, and perhaps carry out functional testing, before making appropriate recommendations.

However, to summarize what we've just covered, here's a simple checklist that you and your practitioner can go through together.

Decode Your Digestion Checklist

Stage 1: The Mouth

- Do you chew your food thoroughly (around 20 times per mouthful)?

- Do you take a break between mouthfuls of food?

- Do you eat in a calm, relaxed environment (i.e. not at your desk while working)?

- Is your nervous system calm and relaxed while you're eating?

Stage 2: The Stomach

- If you have stomach issues, have you been checked for hiatus hernia, gastric ulcers, gastritis, H. pylori infection, stomach cancer, and pernicious anemia?

- Do you have sufficient levels of hydrochloric acid and digestive enzymes?

Stage 3: The Small Intestine

- Do you have signs of a leaky gut, such as brain fog or food intolerances?

- Do you get bloated after eating? Have you been checked for small intestinal bacterial overgrowth (SIBO) or gut dysbiosis?

Stage 4: The Large Intestine

- If you have ongoing issues, ensure you've been considered for inflammatory bowel disease (IBD), diverticulosis, appendicitis, bowel tumors, and Crohn's disease (which can occur anywhere in the digestive tract).

- Do you have pets or work with animals, or have you swum in untreated water (or visited a country with it), where you may have been exposed to parasites?

- Do you pass a 'formed' (not runny, but not hard) stool with ease at least once a day, or do you have issues with either constipation or diarrhea, or both?

Healing digestive function can be an involved and challenging process, but for many people there can also be easy wins, the simplest of which is often diet; we'll be getting into this in much more detail in Chapter 16. But now, it's time to turn our attention to your next bodily system – your hormones. In particular, we're going to explore how your energy reserve system works.

▪▪ Chapter 10 ▪▪

YOUR HORMONES AND YOUR BODY'S ENERGY RESERVE SYSTEM

When Karen first came to The Optimum Health Clinic, she was feeling pretty desperate. Her fatigue wasn't so debilitating that she could no longer function, and she was just about managing her busy life as a mother, homemaker, and part-time interior designer, but in some ways, she wondered if this made things worse.

I remember Karen saying to me, 'If I was as sick as some of your other patients I'd have no choice but to stop.' There was some truth in that – when our fatigue isn't severe, we can sometimes suffer even more because we're able to hang on, and the cycle of suffering is perpetuated without getting fully resolved.

As I reviewed Karen's initial questionnaire, one thing that jumped out at me was her response to a question about food and lifestyle. Karen was consuming an average of five cups of coffee per day; she was eating sugary snacks multiple times a day; and when she became really desperate she relied on 'energy drinks' to keep going. In fact, at least once every few hours, her body was getting another hit of some kind of stimulant.

When I quizzed Karen about her intake of the various stimulants she was using, her response was one I've heard many times: 'It's not that I particularly like coffee or chocolate – I just need the energy hits to get through the day. Without them, I can't function.'

What Karen was describing is a common vicious cycle that many people get into – the more fatigued they become, the more they depend on stimulants to keep them going, and then the more deeply fatigued they become. To understand what was really going on for Karen, we need to take a dive into the way that our hormones, particularly our adrenal hormones, work.

The Body's Energy Reserve System

If you think back to Chapter 3, where we explored the role of your mitochondria, you'll recall that we discussed your body's core energy supply. What we didn't talk about is the many ways this can fluctuate at different points in the day. The factor determining the moment-to-moment, hour-to-hour balance of your energy levels is your hormones.

Think of it like this... The amount of energy our system needs in any given moment will vary greatly – if we're sitting at our desk working quietly or relaxing on the sofa, we're likely to need a small amount of energy, but if we're in the hot seat during an intense meeting, or working out at the gym, our energy need will be considerably higher.

The responsibility for unlocking this extra energy falls in part to your adrenals – two small triangular glands that live on top of each kidney. As well as helping regulate your metabolism and your blood pressure, your adrenal glands are responsible for your body's response to stress. When under stress, your adrenals will release hormones such as cortisol and adrenaline, which cause the temporary upsurge in fuel release/ energy that your body needs in order to respond in that moment.

As Karen discovered, a vicious cycle tends to go on with our adrenal glands – the more fatigued we become, the harder they have to work (see diagram). We then do what we can to boost our energy. Excessive exercise, sugar, caffeine, 'energy drinks,' or whatever else we can get our hands on, will give us a short-term hit of 'energy,' but it's not real energy, and later, we'll pay a price.

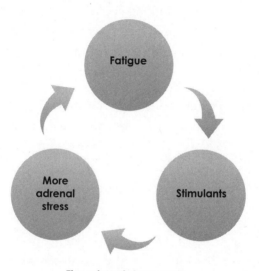

The adrenal stress cycle

The consequence of this reliance on stimulants is that we also create a blood glucose or energy roller coaster that requires our adrenals to step in consistently to offer balance and support. Over time, this places undue pressure on the adrenals, and we start to notice signs of suboptimal adrenal function and associated fatigue.

Yes, you read that right – overuse of anything that provides a short-term boost to your adrenals can make your fatigue symptoms worse, not better, in the long term. That's not to say these things don't have their place; however, depending on them as an energy source can itself be a direct cause of fatigue.

Adrenal Fatigue – What's in a Name?

Some of you may be aware that there is an ongoing debate around the term 'adrenal fatigue.' This has arisen as a result of literature reviews finding inconsistent evidence for reduced hormone output (in particular, cortisol) in fatigue sufferers.[112]

For context, the way we're talking about 'adrenal fatigue' here serves as a simplified metaphor for observing, explaining, and supporting the rebalancing of what's known as your hypothalamic pituitary adrenal axis (HPA).[113, 114]

To be clear, there is a major difference between the subtler functional adrenal *impact* we're discussing here and actual, medically diagnosed adrenal *disease*, such as Addison's disease and Cushing's disease. (Addison's disease is where the adrenals are simply not able to produce enough cortisol, and Cushing's disease is when there is a significant overproduction of cortisol.)

What I'm referring to here is a *functional* difference in adrenal hormones. Put another way: a difference that affects our day-to-day functioning. However, these functional differences can have an enormous impact on our quality of life. To have a sustainable level of energy, we need to support healthy adrenal glands and overall HPA function. Indeed, this brings us to the eighth step in the 12-step plan:

Step 8: Balance your hormones

Six Ways to Balance Your Hormones

To balance your hormones, you have to approach the issue from multiple levels; if you don't do this, you're making the job much more difficult.

1: Reduce Your Stress Burden

The first step is to remove the external stresses that are triggering adrenal spikes in the first place. Hopefully this has already become abundantly clear to you after reading the last few chapters, where we've explored the impact of loads and the fact that for your body to heal, it has to be in a healing state.

If we fail to do this, our adrenals are still being triggered by and having to respond to new stressors – despite everything else we might be doing. I don't want to labor the point, but if you've skipped through the previous chapters, now might be a good time to go back and read them!

2: Remove Stimulants

As we saw in Karen's story above, there is a temptation to use short-term stimulants to compensate for our low adrenal function. The problem with this is that we're creating a fake energy lift, which means an even worse crash will hit us down the line, along with a deepening of our overall fatigue issue. Using any of the following things as a temporary energy source is likely making the situation much worse:

- Caffeine

- Sugar

- Energy drinks (which contain both of the above)

- Recreational drugs

- Excessive carbohydrates, particularly refined carbohydrates

To phase these elements out of our diet and lifestyle, we might need to go gently and wean ourselves off them gradually. But the exhaustion we feel may well be information from our body telling us the reality of where we currently are, and listening to this information can be the first step toward healing; we'll get into this in Part III, where we'll create your plan for recovery.

3: Balance Your Blood Sugar

We'll be getting into diet more in Chapter 16; however, first there is an important point I need to make – the balance of macronutrients on your plate (i.e. protein, fats, and carbohydrates) can have a significant impact on your blood glucose stability, otherwise known as your blood sugar levels – the amount of glucose (sugar) in the blood.

Your blood sugar levels are responsible for maintaining your energy levels. When your blood sugar levels are out of balance, it's the job of your adrenals to work hard to bring back balance. In the box below is a slightly more technical explanation.

▪ ▪ Blood Sugar Explained ▪ ▪

Our blood sugar (glucose) levels should remain within a certain optimal range for health, and we release two hormones, insulin and glucagon, to help maintain healthy blood sugar levels.

The carbohydrates we eat are broken down into glucose molecules, which are absorbed into the bloodstream. When the body detects raised blood sugar (glucose) levels, the pancreas releases the hormone insulin. Insulin shuttles the glucose from our blood into our cells to provide energy, and stores the rest in our muscles, fat cells, and liver for use later.

If our blood sugar level then falls below optimal levels the body releases glucagon, which can release stored glucose back into the bloodstream. This process keeps our blood sugar levels in balance. If our blood sugar rises rapidly, especially after eating a large carbohydrate-based meal, the pancreas can over-react and produce too much insulin.

Our blood sugar (glucose) then takes a rapid, uncomfortable drop, and it may end up too low for normal functioning, which is known as hypoglycemia.[115] This can cause an array of symptoms, including sugar cravings, excess sweating, dizziness, tiredness (fatigue), blurred vision, trembling or shakiness, a fast pulse or palpitations, irritability, difficulty concentrating, and confusion, and it can also cause a release of stress hormones.

Over time, the body can become less sensitive to the effects of insulin, despite the fact that it produces more and more to try to maintain balanced blood sugar levels. This can be especially common in those who are overweight. Eventually, the pancreas may not be able to produce enough insulin to regulate blood sugar levels, leading to hyperglycemia in the long term, which may lead to diabetes.[116]

Blood sugar-balancing habits that help to stabilize levels can be incorporated into our daily routine. They include eating regular meals, avoiding stimulants, including protein, fiber, and healthy fats with every meal, and eating foods with a low GI (Glycemic Index) value.[117] The Glycemic Index is a measure that shows us the impact of a particular food on blood sugar levels.

4: Heal Your Gut

In the last chapter we discussed some of the potential triggers for gastrointestinal inflammation – these include immune reactivity, food intolerances, bacterial imbalance, and the presence of parasites or SIBO. Inflammation in the gut may then result in increased intestinal permeability or a 'leaky gut.'

When we experience gastrointestinal inflammation, the hormone cortisol may be deployed to help mitigate it and offer anti-inflammatory support – the greater the inflammatory burden, the greater the need for cortisol and the greater the pressure on the adrenal glands. This vicious cycle may result in fatigued adrenals and subsequent suboptimal anti-inflammatory support – which of course just perpetuates the inflammatory cycle.

By supporting and improving our digestive health, and reducing our overall inflammation levels, we reduce the burden on our adrenals and cortisol output, which gives them a chance to rebalance. This extra adrenal capacity can also then result in greater capacity in the body to reduce inflammation and attend to the many other roles that the adrenals have functionally, including supporting metabolism and energy production.

This is also a great example of the interconnected nature of recovering from fatigue – when we repair and rebalance one area, it often has an impact on other areas.

5: Balance your Circadian Rhythms

How does your body know how much of its different hormones to release at different points in the day? For example, in healthy adrenal function our cortisol levels should be at their highest in the morning and then gradually reduce as the day continues.[118] Inversely, our melatonin levels (melatonin is the hormone that tells our body it's time to sleep) should be at their lowest in the morning, increase in the evening as we prepare for bed, and hold a long peak through the very early hours of the morning, from around 2 until 5 a.m.[119–121]

Well, these changes are a product of our circadian rhythms, the natural processes that control the body's numerous cycles throughout the day. Factors that influence our circadian rhythms include our mealtimes, exercise timing, and sleep times. A particularly important one is the amount of sunlight going into our eyes at different points in the day, which is a direct communication to our hormone production.

If you think back to our caveman days, during the day we were highly active – we needed to hunt, make shelters, and protect ourselves and our families from the endless threats provided by nature. That meant being alert, and ready for action. As the sun rose in the sky in the morning, the human body evolved to wake up and cue cortisol elevation and melatonin reduction.

Equally, to heal and restore and be ready for action the next day, we needed to wind down and rest deeply at night. The only source of light available to us was fire, which could bring its own risk of alerting predators to our presence, so the human body evolved to switch off at night as darkness came – and once again, this job fell to our hormones.[122] The arrival of darkness cued an increase in melatonin and a reduction in cortisol.

In today's world our circadian rhythms, which have been hundreds of thousands of years in development, have been utterly disrupted by constant light exposure through the evening. Humans have lived on Earth for around 250,000 years, and Thomas Edison's world-changing electric light bulb was only invented 150 years ago – evolutionarily, that's only a moment in our genetic history, and it takes far longer than that for the human body to learn to adapt.

And it's not just light bulbs that are messing with our hormone production and circadian rhythms. What do the majority of us do in the evenings? That's right, we watch television, we read phone screens, we stare at tablets. Indeed, the last thing many people do before they sleep is look at their phone. The impact of the blue light generated by electronic devices directly reduces our production of melatonin.[123-126]

If you think about it, this change in our behavior is only a few decades old. It can take as long as a million years for a species to adjust genetically to a change in its environment, so although our technology may be evolving at an exponential rate, our biology certainly isn't.

All this means that to balance our hormones, we also have to support our circadian rhythms. We need to consider getting a decent amount of sunlight during the day, ideally toward the start of the day, and staying away from too much exposure to artificial light, particularly too much screen time, in the evenings.

Breaking the habit of overusing devices is often not an easy one, but it's essential for our health and that of our loved ones. Research has found that circadian misalignment caused by chronic exposure to artificial light in the evenings may have negative effects on psychological, cardiovascular, and/or metabolic functions.[127, 128]

Blue light from screens disturbs melatonin secretion and affects our internal body clocks, even if the light isn't bright.[129, 130] And, so as to really make the point of just how important honoring our circadian rhythms is, research has shown that short-term night-shift work mimics aspects of chronic fatigue syndrome in one's hormone levels.[131]

So, to help support your adrenals, you need to get enough direct sunlight, particularly in the morning, and avoid excessive use of screens and artificial light in the evening, particularly in the hour before going to sleep. Wearing blue light-blocking glasses in the evening can also help with this.

6: Support Your Adrenals

Although all of the above are critical, when the impact on the adrenals is more severe, they're not always enough on their own. There are a number of additional supports that can be used – although I believe it's very important this isn't done without appropriate supervision from a qualified functional-medicine-trained practitioner, and often with lab tests to confirm the need. What works for someone is a very individual thing, and sometimes we need to experiment with different products, in varying doses, to find the right formula.

The main categories of support are:

- Vitamins and minerals such as Vitamin C, magnesium, and pantothenic acid

- Herbs such as rhodiola, ashwagandha, lemon balm, and l-theanine

- Glandular supplements that offer bovine origin adrenal extracts

- Bio-identical hormones, which have the same structure as naturally occurring endogenous hormones and therefore, courtesy of a 'lock and key' hormone receptor system, can confer health benefits

■ ■ A Note on the Thyroid ■ ■

For the sake of simplicity, and my intention to keep this book as accessible as possible for the lay reader, I've neglected to explore another key aspect of our endocrine system, which is the thyroid.

The thyroid also plays a critically important role in our body's metabolism. There is certainly a subgroup of fatigue sufferers, particularly women, who may also suffer with an underactive thyroid, and this in itself can have an equally potent impact on energy levels.

An underactive thyroid is more likely to be picked up by conventional medical testing than adrenal issues (though not always), but as will perhaps not be a surprise to you now, given our journey together, it isn't best treated by simply ingesting lots of thyroid hormones (although they have their place). Indeed, this can sometimes cause more problems than it solves. As always, an integrative approach like the one we're exploring together, targeting the problem on multiple levels, is still critical.

Turning Vicious Cycles into Virtuous Cycles

As we touched on earlier, there are various vicious cycles in which one area weakens another. For example, reduced cortisol output may result in a lack of systemic anti-inflammatory support, leading to an increased total inflammatory burden, which may in turn increase damage to the mitochondria; this may then negatively impact on energy production and therefore increase fatigue.

Before we move on, I want to make an important point. Just as we can get into vicious cycles where, for example, our reduced cortisol output is affecting the inflammation in our digestive system, which then further reduces our overall energy, and so on, we can also get into virtuous cycles.

Indeed, a key part of our goal is to address some of the lower hanging fruit in your healing journey – to set off a self-perpetuating trend in a positive direction. For example, perhaps you can begin by reducing your use of stimulants and not looking at your phone in the later evening. This means you'll sleep better and wake up feeling more rested. You're then more likely to be out getting some morning light, which will result in a gradual improvement in your morning energy.

You then start eating better, as you have more energy to do so. This helps improve your digestion, which reduces your inflammation. Before you know it, you really don't want or need those stimulants anyway.

Remember, we don't need to change everything at once – far from it. What we need to do is shift the trajectory with manageable and effective changes. Talking of which, it's time to explore our final bodily system – we're going to discuss the impact of your immune system on your energy. To set the frame, we're going to look at one of the biggest medical sagas of the last decade.

■■ Chapter 11 ■■

YOUR IMMUNE SYSTEM – REDUCING YOUR BODY'S LOAD

It was an early morning in October 2009 and as I sat at the desk in my home office reading my most recent emails it was still dark outside. There were more than a dozen relating to the same subject, and when I looked at my phone, I saw that multiple text messages on that topic had arrived overnight.

The previous day, what appeared to be a landmark study had been published in the journal *Science*; it suggested that an infectious agent called xenotropic murine leukemia virus-related virus (XMRV) was a possible explanation for chronic fatigue syndrome.

The study's authors claimed to have detected XMRV in more than 75 percent of 101 patients with chronic fatigue syndrome, and the inference was clear – they believed they'd found a single cause of chronic fatigue syndrome.

Clearly, it was a big story – it was all over the mainstream news, and people were beginning to ask me for comment. However, as I read through the original paper, something felt off to me. Although it was hard to argue with the findings, they just didn't fit with my personal or professional experience.

As the sun came up, I started drafting a public response from The Optimum Health Clinic. I chose my words carefully, but privately I had a feeling that things weren't going to turn out well. Initially, I wondered if something was up with the recruitment of the participants and by a wild coincidence they'd somehow all been exposed to XMRV. However, after further investigation, this seemed unlikely.

In the months that followed, particular pockets of the fatigue community used the findings of the study to reignite a quite unhelpful mind versus body debate. They claimed that the discovery of XMRV in CFS patients was effectively 'evidence' that approaches such as ours, which work with the body and the mind, are clearly incorrect, and I was disappointed to read some quite ugly comment threads in chat rooms.

Just over two years later, in December 2011, the story started to unravel in rather spectacular fashion, culminating in the full retraction of the findings by *Science*. The notice from the journal read, 'Multiple laboratories, including those of the original authors, have failed to reliably detect xenotropic murine leukemia virus-related virus (XMRV) or other murine leukemia virus (MLV)-related viruses in chronic fatigue syndrome (CFS) patients. In addition, there is evidence of poor quality control in a number of specific experiments in the report.'

In the years since, Dr. Judith Mikovits, one of the study's authors, has been discredited even further; researchers have showed that XMRV was created accidentally in the lab during mouse experiments. In essence, it may never have infected any humans. Dr. Mikovits's reputation was in tatters, and more recently she's become a leading voice in support of harmful conspiracy theories surrounding COVID-19.[132]

I think this sad and cautionary tale has something very important to teach us. When something seems 'too good to be true,' it usually is. Furthermore, fatigue is a complex condition that affects different people in different ways, and it'll never be reduced to a single pathogen.

So, although I don't believe we'll ever find that a single pathogen causes the majority of cases of fatigue, overloads to our immune system can have a major impact. For some people a viral infection is the 'straw that breaks the camel's back,' or in our language, the final load. For others, the ongoing load on their immune system has been at the heart of their gradually weakening overall energy, and until the burden is reduced, their body just doesn't have a chance to fight back on its own.

This bring us to the ninth of our steps:

Step 9: Support your immune system

In order to understand the relationship between your immune load and fatigue, I think it's helpful to be aware that your immune system is a large and demanding bodily system for your body to run. This means it uses up a lot of your body's resources, i.e. your energy. So where chronic, low-level immune activation exists, we can expect to see a resulting fatigue. Indeed, we've all experienced this at points in our life when fighting the common cold. When our immune system's working hard, we feel more tired.

Furthermore, an inflammatory response in our immune system, and the various impacts of this on our body, will also directly impact our mitochondria and energy production.[133] That's right – when our immune system's overloaded, it has a direct impact on our cellular energy production.

Three Things That Overload the Immune System

Although immune impacts in fatigue warrant multiple in-depth books of their own, for the sake of simplicity I'm going to focus on the three most common immune challenges faced by people with fatigue. First we'll explore the impact of viral infections such as glandular fever (Epstein-Barr) and then we'll consider toxic mold, followed by Lyme disease and coinfections.

1: Viral Infections

One in 10 people who become infected with glandular fever, Ross River virus, or Coxiella burnetii are found to develop a set of symptoms that meet the criteria for ME/CFS.[134–137] Other viruses that have been found to play a role in the development of chronic fatigue-like symptoms include human herpesvirus 6[138] and rubella.

Given the seemingly causal nature of the virus, and the natural fit with our friend Louis Pasteur's germ theory, as you'd expect there has been some research into the area. However, the findings have been inconsistent, to say the least, in part due to poor research design.

At the OHC, we've also seen a significant number of people infected by COVID-19 develop ongoing fatigue symptoms, commonly known as long COVID. Typically, fatigue that's been triggered by a virus such as this would be classified as post-viral fatigue syndrome.

And, although we definitely see a subgroup of patients whose fatigue appears to be initiated by a viral trigger, in my experience it's rarely that simple. As we explored in Chapter 7, when we talked about the different loads we experience, the viral trigger is usually just the final straw, rather than the cause itself. When you take a step back, you can normally identify the impact of genetics, personality patterns, loads, a maladaptive stress response and so on.[139–141]

When there are cases of post-viral fatigue as described, we'll still primarily treat them with the overall OHC approach, but we may also add in further interventions to support immunity in a general sense. These strategies may include the following tools:

- Zinc

- Vitamin D and/or sunlight exposure

- Vitamin C

- Colostrum

- Supporting the gut microbiome and secretory IgA levels

- Avoiding dietary elements that deplete the system of important immune-supporting nutrients – such as alcohol and refined sugars

- Implementing good sleep hygiene

- Supporting a reduction in anxiety and the maladaptive stress response

- Encouraging a diet rich in natural, unprocessed foods, with a selection of those foods that are replete in nutrients believed to support the function of the immune system

- Supporting stomach acid levels where required

We may also follow these with more specific immune work and testing to identify particular viral loads, and tailored viral protocols to address them.

2: Toxic Mold

Another area that's gained some significant attention in recent years is the impact of toxic mold. In 2005, US physician Dr. Ritchie Shoemaker published a groundbreaking book, *Mold Warriors*, which helped raise awareness of this easily missed, but at times critical, issue.

Molds are a type of fungus and are present everywhere, including the air that we breathe. When people talk of mold toxicity, they sometimes name the culprit as black mold; however, many molds are black, and what they're actually referring to is a type called Stachybotrys chartarum (S. chartarum), also known as Stachybotrys atra.

Molds tend to thrive in damp indoor environments, and it appears that around 25 percent of the population is sensitive to molds. It's important to understand that certain molds produce toxic compounds called mycotoxins; these can be absorbed through the gut, lungs, and skin, and exposure to them has been associated with CFS symptoms.[142, 143] The impact of mycotoxin exposure can be an extended array of immune-related symptoms.[144, 145] Here are a few of them:

- Sneezing

- Runny or stuffy nose

- Cough and postnasal drip

- Itchy eyes, nose, and throat

- Watery eyes

- Dry, scaly skin

- Elevated histamine levels

- Feeling worse in the autumn months

- Headaches

- Muscular symptoms

- Mood changes

- Brain fog and changes in neurological function[146]

I think it's also helpful to note three rather unusual symptoms that are quite specific to mycotoxin exposure:

- Electric shock sensations

- Ice pick-like pains

- Vibrating or pulsating sensations running up and down the spinal cord

One of the medical practitioners I most respect is Dr. Neil Nathan, and in his excellent book *Toxic: Heal your body from Mold Toxicity, Lyme Disease, Multiple Chemical Sensitivities and Chronic Environmental Illness* he makes the point that if these symptoms are happening alongside our more common fatigue symptoms, 'the possibility of mold toxicity should immediately jump to mind.'

The good news is that it's relatively simple to look for the presence of mycotoxins through functional testing with a suitably qualified practitioner.

3: Lyme Disease and Coinfections

Lyme disease is a bacterial infection caused by being bitten by an infected tick. Although only a small number of ticks are infected with the bacteria that causes Lyme, the disease appears to be on the rise, with the number of cases diagnosed in the USA doubling between 2000 and 2019.[147]

Our understanding of Lyme disease has evolved year on year, but there is still a lot that we don't know.[36] Indeed, there are raging disagreements between conventional medical wisdom and those in the frontline trenches supporting the people affected. Conventional wisdom says that the tick that bites you needs to be latched on for at least 36 hours for the virus to be transmitted and that if you don't experience a bull's-eye-shaped rash afterward then you've likely not been infected. However, in our experience, there are too many anecdotal cases that contradict this for it to hold true.

The situation is further complicated by the fact that standard medical tests for Lyme are not as accurate as some doctors believe.[37] Indeed, they can produce false negatives (people being told they don't have Lyme when they do) for a number of reasons. These include:

- Testing only for the bacteria Borrelia burgdorferi and leaving out many other species, including the recently discovered Borrelia mayonii

- Tests not being sensitive enough

- Tests depend on measuring antibodies, and some people may be slower to produce these, or indeed struggle to do so

- Coinfections complicating the immune picture

If Lyme disease is caught quickly it's much easier to treat; and, along with SIBO, which we discussed in Chapter 9, it's a good example of where antibiotics can have an important role to play. However, many of those bitten by a tick and infected with Lyme disease don't even notice. It's only when they start experiencing symptoms that they realize something's wrong, and that may be months, or even years, later.

Indeed, I've observed many times that although the Lyme has weakened someone's system, it's only when a perfect storm of the other factors we've been exploring comes together that they finally start experiencing symptoms. The Lyme was always having an impact but the gradual effect of this, followed by the overwhelm of other factors, meant the body finally began to lose the battle.

Although symptoms resulting from Lyme disease vary considerably, the majority of those with chronic (ongoing) Lyme will experience fatigue, alongside:

- Achy, stiff, or swollen joints

- Headaches, dizziness and/or fever

- Night sweats and sleep disturbances

- Cognitive decline – i.e. issues with focus and concentration

Thankfully, within the functional medicine community, particularly via Armin Labs in Germany (with whom we work closely), there are tests that give much more reliable information, not only on Lyme disease but also on other coinfections such as Bartonellosis and Babesiosis. Although this testing can be expensive, when it's indicated as necessary it can be a critical step in formulating a plan to move forward.

If diagnosing Lyme disease medically sounds confusing, building a path to recovery can be even more complicated. In recent years there has been an important and ultimately helpful surge of interest in Lyme disease and coinfections, in part due to high-profile sufferers such as the Canadian singer-songwriters Avril Lavigne and Justin Bieber.

However, I've noticed a trend alongside this for people with a previous diagnosis of ME, CFS, or fibromyalgia to disregard that for a confirmed Lyme diagnosis, in the belief that this is a much more accurate diagnosis of a single pathogen invading their body that needs to be nuked.

This is perfectly understandable – not least because it can help shed the cultural stigma of a standard CFS diagnosis – but I notice that people end up throwing the proverbial baby out with the bathwater. Believing that all they need to do is eradicate the Lyme in their system, they ignore all the other key principles we've covered so far in this book.

In my experience, if someone has Lyme, they may well need to use targeted interventions to address it directly; however, without also working to understand their personality patterns, remove other loads, cultivate a healing state, heal their digestion, balance their hormones, and so on, they end up making themselves feel even more unwell with the treatment.

That said, if someone does have Lyme, these other interventions may only take them so far. When it comes to addressing the Lyme and associated coinfections, there are a number of emerging interventions that largely fall into two main categories:

1. **Antimicrobial/herbal protocols** – these are offered by functional health practitioners who'd argue they are more multifaceted and offer a more holistic solution, with each botanical and supplement having a range of effects.

2. **Antibiotic protocols** – these are the intervention of choice for conventional medicine doctors and some integrative medicine doctors, who may use antibiotics in tandem with herbal and nutritional protocols.

The debate around botanical antimicrobials versus pharmaceutical antibiotic approaches for Lyme and coinfections is beyond the scope of this book because it's complex, nuanced, and still emerging. What I will say is that I've seen evidence that both approaches work, and at the OHC we're always careful to help each individual navigate the path forward that's most suitable for them.

Total Immune Load

For some people, the situation is complicated by multiple loads on their immune system; perhaps there is a history of a tick bite and unresolved Lyme disease, and alongside this toxic mold exposure followed by a final trigger of glandular fever.

In such cases, it's important to sequence interventions in the right order. Here, you might first build up the overall immune resilience, then focus on eradicating mycotoxins, and then finally address the immune-related consequences of Lyme and coinfections. The logic for this is that mold is generally easier to test and eradicate, and with this load improved, it becomes easier to then tackle the bacterial and viral load in the body.

Here's a checklist to help you decode the role your immune load could be playing in your fatigue.

The Immune Overload Checklist

To help identify your possible immune loads, consider the following questions:

1. Have you suffered from viral infections such as Epstein-Barr virus (glandular fever), Ross River virus, Coxiella burnetii, or COVID-19?

2. Are you aware of having been exposed to excessive damp or toxic mold? Or are you experiencing electric shock sensations, ice pick-like pains, or vibrating or pulsating sensations running up and down the spinal cord?

3. Have you been bitten by a tick, or any insect, and recall experiencing an inflammatory response in the area of the bite? Or do you have achy, stiff, or swollen joints, particularly where the joint pain is migratory and moves around the body?

In reality, much of what we've been exploring in recent chapters will require you to work with an experienced practitioner, such as those at the OHC. That's even more the case when it comes to supporting immune function. That said, there is a great deal you can do to support yourself, and that's where we're turning our attention now – it's time for us to start devising your path to recovery.

Part III

RECOVERING

FROM

FATIGUE

▪▪ Chapter 12 ▪▪

COACHING YOURSELF
FOR RECOVERY

In Part I we explored a new model for understanding fatigue, and in Part II we looked at the physiological and psycho-emotional elements that are important in helping you decode your fatigue. In this section I want to help you start to create a plan for your healing journey using the second of our fatigue maps: your path to recovery.

However, before we get into the specifics of the recovery map, I think it's important to ensure that you've established the right mindset for rolling it out. My deep hope is that this book is playing a critical role in empowering you to decode your fatigue and to move forward on your healing journey.

For this to be effective, you must become a champion of your own success. That means you need to be able to motivate yourself on your low days, taper your enthusiasm on your good days – so you don't go too fast (which will likely result in an energy crash) – and ultimately, be the one who's there for you when perhaps no one else is. In essence, you need to take on the role of your biggest champion and become your own inner coach.

The 3Ds to Success

As I was cultivating my inner coach in the first few years of my healing journey, I came up with a model called 'The 3Ds to success,' and it's one that I still use with clients today. Here's what the 3Ds are: you need to *Decide* what you want and that you're ready to do whatever it takes; you then need to *Devise* your strategy; and finally, you need to *Do* something and build momentum. In this chapter we're going to drill down into this model in more detail and help you get in the best possible headspace for your healing.

Decide

If you recall from the opening chapter that life-changing conversation I had with my uncle, you'll know that the critical turning point in my own healing was the realization that if I wanted the circumstances of my life to change, I would need to be the one to change them.

Ultimately, it all came down to a *decision* – was I going to continue watching my life disappear in front of my eyes or was I going to do whatever it took to turn my life around? What was particularly impactful for me was recognizing that every day I failed to take action, I was unconsciously deciding that my life would stay the same.

One of the things I struggled with at the time of that conversation was the limit of my capacity. I had limited money, very limited knowledge (I was only 18 years old), and although I didn't know it then, I was also enormously limited in terms of access to information (we're talking pre-mass access to the internet!) Who was I to think I'd find answers to an illness that was baffling the world's medical experts?

To challenge these beliefs, my uncle recommended I expose myself to the ideas and beliefs of others who'd faced great adversity and found a way through it. I'd never been much of a reader before then but my uncle persuaded me to start reading biographies; and, with not much else to do, I soon became hooked.

Initially, my uncle would send me books that he thought I might find inspiring, but once I'd got through those, I started visiting the local library and bookshop to seek out more. Even that wasn't an easy step for me – approaching the person at the checkout and telling them I wanted to order books on self-help felt almost more embarrassing than the time in my early teens when my friends dared me to buy a pornographic magazine from the local newsagent.

As I continued to read these books, some of the authors became my heroes. Other teenage boys had posters of sports people or musicians on their walls, but if it'd been possible, I'd have put up posters of those people whose books took me a step closer to the belief that recovery from fatigue was possible. Indeed, it was back then that the seeds were sown for the interviews I've conducted with the dozens and dozens of people who've shared their recovery stories with me over the years.

One of the books that had the biggest impact on me was *My Life and Vision* by Meir Schneider. Meir had been born blind and told there was no way he'd ever be able to see. During his teenage years he became increasingly frustrated by the limits of his life and made the decision that whatever it took, he'd find a way to see. As a teenager on my own healing journey, I found this attitude very inspiring; however, it was what Meir did next that impressed me the most.

He researched everything he could about sight and eventually came across the Bates method of eye exercises for improving eyesight. Some of these exercises involved looking at the sun with closed eyes and repeatedly covering and uncovering the eyes with the palms. If you can imagine being given tedious and boring practices like these, you'd think that sticking to them for just a few minutes a day might be a challenge. Not for Meir – he did these, and various other exercises he discovered, for many hours every single day. His investment in doing whatever it took to heal was extraordinary.

The result? Well, after several years Meir's sight started to develop, and it eventually improved to the point where he was granted a driver's license. For me, the moral of this story was clear: if Meir could find a way to recover his sight, and the factor that made the difference was the level of commitment he brought to the process, I was going to do the same for my own healing.

As I explained in Chapter 1, for the next five years, my recovery became *everything* to me. I meditated and practiced yoga for hours a day; I made radical changes to my eating habits; and at one point I was taking 62 supplements a day (which isn't something I'd recommend anyone do!) And I reached a point where, in some areas, I had an equal level of knowledge with some of the practitioners I was consulting.

Indeed, toward the end of my healing journey I started to work with one practitioner who'd written half a dozen books in the field; I'd read every single one, made detailed notes, and I was consulting her to confirm the nuances of how I'd apply her protocol to my situation.

Become Captain of the Ship of Your Recovery

With this book, my goal isn't that you'll become a leading expert on fatigue. What you do need to become, though, is an expert on your personal manifestation of fatigue. As we'll get into in the next few chapters, you need to learn to listen to your body so you know when it needs you to rest, and when it's ready for a bit of a push. You need to make decisions about which practitioners to see and when, and you need to know when it's time to move on from a particular approach that isn't working – or indeed when to hang in there when everyone around you has lost faith.

I liken this to being the captain of a ship. The ship's captain will most likely know a lot less about engineering than the ship's engineer; he won't be as good a navigator as the navigator; and he almost certainly won't be as good a cook as the chef. However, the captain isn't the captain because he can do everyone else's job better than they can, but because he has the ability to *direct*, and to get the best out of, each of those specialists.

To become captain of the ship of your recovery, you do need to be informed and books like this, along with its companion course (access this at www.alexhoward.com/fatigue) play a key role. You also need to learn to understand the language of your body because this will offer critical feedback while navigating along the way. We'll be getting to that next.

Put bluntly – if you want your life to be different, and if you want to reclaim your energy, you're going to have to *decide* that this is more important than many other things in your life. The journey may also be challenging at times, and you'll need to be prepared for that.

Devise

Once you've decided that your recovery is going to become one of the most important things in your life, and that you're going to give everything to it, you then need to *devise* a strategy for moving forward, using this book as a foundation.

But while we're on the subject, here's a word of caution: be careful not to get sucked into analysis paralysis. Although the landscape for learning around fatigue has changed radically in the quarter-century since I first became ill and made my nervous trips to the local library and bookshop, you could argue that we now have almost the opposite problem. My issue was that there was very little information out there, whereas the challenge today is that there is too much. Knowing where to start when your body is sensitive, and your time and money are limited, can be very challenging.

The danger is that we end up in a state of analysis paralysis – we have so much data and so many conflicting opinions flying around in our head that we just don't know where to begin. And the truth is that you *do* have to start somewhere.

Work Out How to Move Forward

To break the deadlock of analysis paralysis when it comes to weighing up a given approach to fatigue, I encourage you to ask yourself the following questions:

1. Is it logical and does it make sense in your mind?

2. Does it feel intuitively right to you?

3. Does this path fit with your previous experiences?

4. Is there evidence that this path has worked for others in a similar situation?

If you can satisfy these questions, then often it's better to start somewhere than to wait endlessly in analysis.

Let's say that someone's enthusiastically promoting a certain approach to you – it worked for them and they're evangelical about it, However, it simply doesn't make sense to you, or for your situation. In this instance, I'd say listen to your own instincts, not theirs. Or perhaps something *does* make sense to you – it might even feel intuitively right – but it simply doesn't fit with your own previous experiences. Again, that's something you should listen to.

I remember one patient whose recovery journey was especially complex and challenging. Monica's body, for reasons that are still not fully understood, used the thyroid hormone T3 in a very particular way that made her crash severely whenever she stopped taking it. The dose she needed to balance her levels and reduce her symptoms was expensive, and it didn't entirely follow conventional wisdom. To put it in medical terms, she was atypical.

So, each time Monica went to a new endocrinologist, the first thing they did was try and reduce her dose, or even get her to go cold turkey. They'd tell her that the claims she was making about her body couldn't be true because they weren't backed by science – essentially, they were saying that the science was right and her body was wrong. However, the fact remained that every time Monica's dose was reduced, she'd crash again and would need at least six months to recover.

When I'm working alongside other practitioners, I try to 'stay in my lane' and respect their professional decisions; however, in this case, the pattern eventually became so painfully obvious – particularly to Monica, who was going through hell each time – that I could no longer hold my tongue. I spent a session working with Monica, building up her confidence to go back to her GP and not only demand the medicine that was critical to her quality of life but also advocate for her own truth, regardless of the fact that science hadn't yet caught up with it.

When it comes to devising your path to recovery, you have to be a willing and active participant. You have to take responsibility for the decisions you make, and only you can truly be the one to advocate for yourself and your needs. But in the end, you've got to start somewhere.

Do

Once you've decided to become captain of the ship of your recovery, and you've devised your plan to start moving forward, it's time to act. It's time to *do* something. After all, knowledge is nice but it's action that creates change. And to take that action, you need to believe that it's possible for someone to heal from fatigue – and that it's possible for *you* to do so. Ultimately, you need to have the right beliefs.

The Power of Belief

There is plenty of data on beliefs and their power. If you think about it, the single most researched drug in modern medicine is the power of belief, or to use its scientific term, placebo. Every single drug that's given a license has to be tested against the power of an inert placebo, to ensure the 'effects' of the drug are more than someone's expectation that it will help them.

Belief, or placebo, can in some cases have all kinds of miraculous effects on the body; indeed, the way this power can be unlocked has been the subject of many books. However, in my opinion, there is a very simple and practical mechanism in which belief is important – if we don't believe that something's going to be effective, we're unlikely to invest the time, money, and energy in finding out.

For example, when we're put on a new supplement program, if we don't believe it's going to help us, we're unlikely to make the effort to remember to take the supplements. If we reflect on Meir Schneider's extraordinary feat of regaining his eyesight, we'll realize that at the core of his dedication to practicing those exercises was the belief that they *could* work.

Start With Hope

It can sometimes feel impossible to go from where we are now to the belief that something's going to work, especially when we've little evidence for it. If the top of the table is the belief that recovery is possible, then the legs that support that tabletop are the evidence. Right now, you might not have many legs for that table, and they might not be that strong; this means that your starting point is to begin gathering that evidence – namely, putting things into action sufficiently that you see some evidence in your own experience, and actively focusing on challenging the beliefs you hold. The more legs you gather for that tabletop, the stronger that belief will become.

Sometimes all we have to start with is hope, and *that* is enough – there is something of a continuum from hoping to believing to *knowing*. The more legs we gather for that tabletop belief, the stronger it becomes; and with enough solid legs, we can know with certainty that we're going to recover.

Positive Action Feeds Positive Action

One of the things I've noticed while working with patients is that sometimes it's hard to get things moving in a new direction. Getting a car from stationary to 10 miles an hour takes a lot more power than getting it from 10 miles an hour to 20. Once the car is moving we have momentum and then it's more about sustaining the movement. The same is true when it comes to activating change in humans.

Getting started can be difficult, but as soon as we begin to see positive changes and we move along the continuum from hoping to believing, the journey does become easier. I think the trick is to set up the game so we can win. If you put in place some of the easier changes in this book, and gather evidence that they're working, the more challenging changes will then feel more achievable. We'll get more into that in Chapter 18.

Toxic Positivity

One note of caution on beliefs, though: much has been written in popular psychology about the importance of having positive thoughts, controlling our mind, not being negative, and so on. And although I very much believe we need to become captain of the ship of our own recovery, I'm not a believer in unrealistic positive thinking. My experience is that what goes up in a way that's unsupported, comes crashing back down again in time. Consider shares on the stock market – if something shoots up due to unsubstantiated hype, it's almost guaranteed to crash back down.

The same is true on the healing journey: if we try to convince ourselves that we have more energy than we do, eventually we're going to run out, and that means a crash. This is something we'll discuss a lot more in the next chapter.

Recently, people have started using the phrase 'toxic positivity' to refer to focusing only on the positive and rejecting and negating the 'negative' of our experience, which I think captures this pattern perfectly. Just as chemical toxicity is poisonous to our body, constantly seeing things differently to how they are causes endless suffering and is a poison for the mind and heart.

I believe strongly in seeing things as they actually are; however, because many fatigue sufferers have been consistently exposed to the factually inaccurate opinions of the conventional medical world, which insist that fatigue is either in the mind or is incurable, they can become overly negative as a form of self-protection.

When we shift from being negative to being *realistic*, this might appear to be positive thinking to some, but as long as our ideas are grounded in reality we're in the right place. When you do my job for long enough, you realize that fatigue is absolutely a condition from which we can heal; however, as we're exploring in this book, we first need to decode what's going on and then carefully map a path that works.

Commitment vs. Surrender

Although there is no question that consistent, considered action is a critical ingredient for the healing journey, we do also have to be careful to maintain a balance. A significant trap that people fall into – it's certainly one to which I succumbed – is using the same strategies that caused them to become ill in the first place to try and turn things around.

Effectively, we get fatigued in part because of our achiever pattern and pushing ourselves too hard; we then attempt to apply the same strategy to the healing journey. However, as we'll discuss further in the next chapter, you can't push your way to recovery. You also can't just do nothing and rest your way to recovery. You have to decode your fatigue, put together the right plan, and then *heal* your way to recovery.

It's a balance between having the *commitment* to be disciplined enough to do the things that need to be done, and having the ability to *surrender* – to let go, trust, and cultivate a healing state in the body. This balance is different for different people at different times, but both qualities are important.

If we've spent a lifetime mastering ways to push through limitations and override the communications and feedback from our body, then our biggest challenge may well be to learn to trust and surrender. Remember what we discussed back in Chapter 5 – the question isn't necessarily what *caused* us to get sick but what's *stopping* us from healing. Pushing our recovery too hard is definitely an example of the latter.

So, to summarize the main points in this chapter:

- You need to *decide* that you're going to make healing your body one of the most important things in your life.

- Next, you need to *devise* a plan to get there.

- Finally, you need to *do* something – you need to take action.

In Chapter 18 we'll work together to create your recovery plan. But before we do, you need to understand how to listen to your body and to gauge how much activity you should be doing.

■■ Chapter 13 ■■

LEARNING TO LISTEN
TO YOUR BODY

'**Y**ou'll feel better if you get some exercise.'

'It's probably just depression – stop thinking about it and get on with things.'

'We all get tired sometimes, so stop complaining and push on with life.'

This is the kind of 'advice' that's routinely aimed at people suffering from fatigue. Although the words might vary, the message is the same: ignore your body, push through, and you'll feel better. It's one thing when it comes from well-intentioned family members – although it hurts, it's generally easier to dismiss – but it's another when the medical professionals we trust to know what they're talking about use the very same words. If *they* tell us to push through, then the chances are we'll at least try to do so.

But where does this position come from? It must be based on some kind of research, right? With so many millions of people suffering so severely, such a potentially harmful approach must be based in real evidence. Well, yes, it is... but things aren't quite as they seem.

The PACE trial – a Medical Scandal

In 2011 a paper was published in the respected British medical journal *The Lancet* that shared the findings of one of the largest ever studies into ME/CFS.[148] The PACE trial randomized 641 participants into a four-armed study looking at cognitive behavior therapy (CBT), graded exercise therapy (GET), adaptive pacing therapy (APT), and specialist medical care (SMC).

In the UK, CBT and GET are used in conventional medicine for working with chronic fatigue syndrome. The underlying premise of both approaches is that fatigue is effectively a state of deconditioning in the body and that the sufferer has become habituated to feeling tired; by changing unhelpful thought patterns and reconditioning the body, a path to recovery can be found. In essence, the hidden assumption is that the fatigue isn't biological in nature, and changes in behavior will help the sufferer realize this.

In the trial, it was claimed that 12 months after randomization, two of the therapies, cognitive behavior therapy (CBT) and graded exercise therapy (GET), were more effective in improving both patient-reported fatigue and physical functioning than either adaptive pacing therapy (APT) or specialist medical care (SMC) alone.

Indeed, the PACE trial concluded that 59 percent of chronic fatigue syndrome patients receiving CBT and 61 percent receiving GET had improved, and an accompanying editorial suggested that 22 percent of patients had recovered. As a result of this finding, CBT and GET have become the treatments of choice for fatigue in the UK, along with the idea that our body is wrong and should be ignored.

The PACE trial was publicly funded by the UK's Medical Research Council, the Department for Work and Pensions, the Department of Health for England, and the Scottish Chief Scientific Office, with a combined cost of almost £5 million. You'd certainly be forgiven for thinking that the respected organizations behind the study, the involvement of a leading scientific journal, and the meaningful sample size indicates that these findings are of significant value to the fatigue community, but in fact, you'd be dangerously wrong.

As a result of some outstanding work by Dr. Sarah Myhill, and other leading figures in the UK's ME/CFS community, the credibility of the PACE trial has been systematically dismantled at every level.[149, 150] The following are just some of their findings:

- The level of change needed to determine improvement was lowered after the trial had begun.

- The kind of strict sampling expected in a trial of this nature was not used.

- Bias was introduced by promoting the success of the interventions to participants (i.e. creating a possible placebo response).

- Some of the trial team were also reviewers of the paper (which totally undermines the process of peer review).

- Initial gains reported at the end of the trial mostly disappeared at follow-up; this was not reported.

- Objective tests of physical function were not generally used, only self-reporting of outcomes by participants; this means they were really measures of mood rather than actual physical function.

I think the most striking finding was that when the correct research measures were applied, two-thirds of the claimed improvement disappeared. We only know any of this to be the case because, after a lengthy legal battle, the raw data was released so it could be reanalyzed. The resulting war of words continues to this day.[151, 152]

The Impact of Bad Science

Without pointing any fingers, I think that in a situation like this one has to follow the money somewhat and look at who funded the study. CBT and GET are cheap, short-term therapies that can be administered relatively easily. And perpetuating the narrative that ME/CFS are not real physical illnesses allows the UK's Department for Work and Pensions to continue to refuse disability payments to those most in need.

Personally, I don't think it's possible to exaggerate the damage done by this research, and other studies like it, and I'm far from alone in this view.[153, 154] It's not only the impact of utterly incorrect advice, which causes people constantly to push through, do too much, and therefore become more severely fatigued; such research also fuels the cultural misunderstandings around fatigue and the idea that it's all in the mind. This leads to disbelief and cynicism about the validity of our condition from family and friends – the very people we should be able to go to for emotional support.

The heart of the matter is, if you suffer from fatigue and you've spoken to conventional medicine professionals, you've likely been encouraged to push through, and to see your body's communications as flawed on some level; ultimately, you've been given the message that you need to stop feeling sorry for yourself and just get on with it. However, this is literally the *opposite* of what you should be doing.

If I'm saying that pushing through and ignoring your body is the opposite of what you should be doing, what does that mean? Should you just do nothing and wait until you feel like you have energy? Maybe, but not necessarily, and we'll get into that. The headline is: fatigue is real and you can't push yourself better. And often, you can't just do nothing and rest yourself better. What you need to do is *heal* yourself better. You need to address the underlying physical and psycho-emotional issues; you need to calm your nervous system; and everything else we've talked about so far. But let's now look at how much activity you should do.

How Do You Listen to Your Body?

To answer this question for yourself, you're going to have to learn a new language – the language of listening to your body. As with learning any new language, you're going to make plenty of mistakes along the way and will have to be gentle with yourself during the process.

You see, the human body has extraordinary wisdom, and it's attempting to communicate with us all of the time. From the more obvious things such as hunger telling us we need to eat, to sleepiness telling us we need to sleep, the body is constantly giving us messages. The question isn't whether the messages are there, but whether we're actually listening to them.

If we've spent a lifetime learning to override and ignore our body, then learning to slow down, listen to it, and decipher its communications will take time. And the situation isn't made easier by the fact that it's rarely one communication – often, our body is saying a whole load of contradictory things simultaneously, and our job is to decipher all of this and figure out what we need to do with it.

I liken this job to being the chairman in a board meeting. You have the marketing director saying he needs more budget for advertising and giving a rosy view of what's coming down the sales funnel. You then have the finance director, who's concerned about cash flow and wants to cut spending. The CEO is focused toward the company vision and how to navigate the different trends and opportunities coming down the line in the sector. The chairman's job is to listen to everyone on the board and to help guide the discussion toward considered and strategic decision making.

It's the same with your body. Your energy levels tell you that you need to rest and do less; your mind is stressing about the work assignment that's a week overdue; your inner child is feeling frustrated and wants to have a blow-out and go party with your friends; the rational part of you says to take it one step at a time; and your anxiety pattern tells you it's all hopeless anyway. It's no wonder you feel confused!

The situation is only made more challenging by the fact that the messages from our body change over time, and they're unique to each individual. Although a skillful practitioner with a lot of experience of working with fatigue patients can help you interpret and decipher your body's communications, it's far from a perfect science, and they're still partly relying on your ability to relay what your body's telling you.

So the first step in learning to listen to your body means doing just that – listening. Not getting angry with your body, not pushing it, not trying to coax it into doing a bit more. No – really, truly, honestly listening. When you do that, how does your body actually feel?

This is one of the fundamental ways in which the OHC's approach is so different to traditional adaptive pacing therapy. With traditional pacing, you decide on a baseline and how you'll increase it based on a predetermined plan. With the OHC approach, we're getting out of your mind and into your body, and letting it be the master. Put another way, traditional pacing tells your body what it should be doing, while the OHC approach lets your body tell you.

Questions to Ask When Listening to Your Body

Here are some of the questions I ask my patients as a way to better focus their attention on listening to their body:

1. When you do a particular activity, does it give you more energy or less?

2. Do you have to keep pushing yourself to get through your daily routine? Or, if you stay connected and listening to your body, does your energy level stay constant?

3. When you go to bed at night, do you feel as if you still have a little energy left in the tank? Or are you totally spent?

4. When you wake in the morning, do you feel like getting up, or do you have to force yourself to do so?

The Four Types of Tiredness

In the early years of the OHC, while helping patients better listen to their body, my friend and colleague Anna Duschinsky noticed that all tiredness is not the same. Indeed, she identified four different types of tiredness, each with its own causes and with different strategies effective in helping resolve it. This model, which we've come to call the 'four types of tiredness,' is both incredibly simple and immensely helpful.

Type 1: Mental Tiredness

This is when the mind is overtired.

Signs and Causes

Signs of mental tiredness can be struggling to find words, brain fog, mental confusion, or a sense that our mind is overstimulated and unable to settle. Mental tiredness is often caused by an anxiety pattern pushing our mind into overdrive, and it can also be a product of too much mental effort for our current energy levels.

How to Help It

The best resolution for mental tiredness is to allow your mind to rest by reducing stimulation. Different things will work for different people here – you might find that anything from watching mindless TV shows to listening to podcasts acts as a helpful distraction and allows your mind to settle; or you might find that you need to reduce your exposure to noise and light and simply let your brain have full rest.

Type 2: Emotional Tiredness

This is when you feel emotionally drained.

Signs and Causes

Signs of emotional tiredness are being emotionally sensitive or reactive and feeling at our limit emotionally. We'll often overreact to small things and lack resourcefulness – as if we don't have the emotional capacity to take on anything else. Emotional tiredness is often the result of a helper pattern running to excess.

How to Help It

Taking some time away from the source of our emotional overwhelm is likely important. This may involve setting firmer boundaries with other people; taking uninterrupted time alone; and allowing ourselves to feel into and connect to ourselves emotionally. Ultimately, avoiding our emotions is rarely an effective strategy. To process and digest our emotions, we need to open to and feel them.

Type 3: Physical Tiredness

This is when our physical body is overtired.

Signs and Causes

Signs of physical tiredness are aching muscles and physical weakness – the feeling that all you want to do is lie down and rest. Physical tiredness (beyond the ongoing tiredness of your current condition) is the result of doing too much activity, not listening to your body, and not taking rest when needed. Put another way, it's when your achiever pattern has been out of control.

How to Help It

The key to overcoming physical tiredness is listening to your body and working with your 'baseline,' as we're about to explore. This can sometimes require periods of deep physical rest and working to build up your energy reserves, so you don't run out of energy so quickly when you're active.

Type 4: Environmental Tiredness

Environmental tiredness is when you become tired and drained by a lack of variety in your physical environment. Monotony and repetitiveness of environment can themselves become draining.

Signs and Causes

Signs of environmental tiredness can be less obvious than the other three types of tiredness. They can include a sense of flatness and apathy, feeling drained by small things, and a sense of despondency and hopelessness. In fatigue, the usual cause of environmental tiredness is being limited in energy, and therefore spending increasing amounts of time in the same small space.

How to Help It

If we have the physical energy to do so, changing our environment can have a significant impact on alleviating environmental tiredness. If we can't change the location of our physical environment, changing things *within* the environment can also be helpful – for example, moving furniture around, redecorating a room we've been in for a long time, or something as simple as lighting a scented candle.

Another simple tip is avoiding spending the whole day lying in bed – so if you're housebound or partially bedbound, relocating to the sofa, even for some of the day, can help give you a lift.

It's important to bear in mind that with each of these types of tiredness, when our overall energy is low we'll reach our limits on them more quickly. For example, something like paying some of our bills online, which with a normal level of energy would be a breeze, can quickly lead to mental tiredness if our energy is reduced.

However, one of the very helpful things this model does is enable us to address what we actually need. For example, treating all types of tiredness in the same way, such as with increased physical rest, may not be all that effective. After all, if we have emotional tiredness, spending more hours in bed is not going to replace our need for better boundaries.

Now that we've explored the importance of listening to your body, the next thing we need to look at is what you do with the information you find. You see, although for much of the time your body's going to be telling you it's tired, the chances are you still need to function in your life, even if it's at a very low level.

So, should you rest? Should you do things even when you don't feel like it? Should you follow some kind of structure or routine? Well, the fact is it depends on which stage of recovery you're at, which is what we'll look at in the next chapter.

▪▪ Chapter 14 ▪▪

THE THREE STAGES OF RECOVERY

James was only in his early twenties when he first came to the OHC. He was suffering from debilitating chronic fatigue that left him virtually housebound and almost entirely cut off from his friends and peers. And, like most people whose lives have been torn apart so cruelly, he was angry. He was angry at the doctors who'd let him down, he was angry at his situation, and he was angry that there appeared to be no way out.

Personally, I don't subscribe to much of the popular psychology language around positive and negative emotions; of course, throwing our anger out at the world often just causes more hurt, but at the core of the emotion of anger is our personal power – and that's a power we often need to fuel the difficult path of healing.

For James, one of the key turning points in his recovery was realizing he needed to channel his anger into the rigor of following the plan we helped him come up with, a key ingredient of which was listening to his body. When I interviewed him about his story for our documentary film (which is included in the Decode Your Fatigue companion course), he remarked that 'You wouldn't leave the house with your phone on only a 15 percent charge, and you shouldn't be doing the same with your body.'

As the months unfolded on his journey with the OHC, James became increasingly disciplined about listening to his body. If he didn't have the energy to do an activity he'd planned, he cancelled it. If his body needed him to rest, he rested. When it was time to calm his system, he focused hard on that. Although such rigorous pacing was certainly not the only variable on James's healing path, it was a key foundation for his recovery.

In learning what his body could and couldn't do, James was able to work with it rather than against it. He was able to avoid crashes from doing too much, and along the way, he also cultivated a deep healing state – after all, there is nothing more stressful than constantly battling energy crashes. A significant factor in supporting James with this process was our model of the three stages of recovery.

Which Stage of Recovery Are You At?

One of my biggest breakthroughs in understanding fatigue was the realization that the recovery journey has three different stages. What works at one stage can make things worse at another stage, so identifying which stage you're at, and tailoring your approach and activity accordingly, is absolutely crucial to successful recovery.

In brief, the three recovery stages are the deep rest stage; the tired and wired stage; and the reintegration stage. We tend to go through these stages sequentially, and if we have a relapse we'll often cycle back through them in a much shorter period of time. Let's explore each recovery stage in more detail.

Stage 1: Deep Rest

The deep rest stage is characterized by deep physical exhaustion that's not initially alleviated by sleep or rest. Some people will go into this stage right at the beginning of their fatigue journey – i.e. when there is sudden onset – while others will gradually weaken until they reach this point. Some people will never quite go to this stage, which can be a problem in itself because it's at stage 1 that deep rest and healing should be happening.

Signs That You're In It

The main indicator that we're in stage 1 is that our fatigue is overwhelming. Sleeping more, doing less activity, reducing our social interaction and so on can be very important, but initially it may feel as if these measures are having little impact (although it's most likely that they are).

How to Move Through It

When we're at this stage, it's critical to get as much deep physical rest as we can. Sometimes, the depth of the exhaustion we feel can be quite terrifying, but the more we try to fight it or ignore it, the harder this stage can become. No amount of pushing through at this stage works; indeed, it almost always makes things worse. At stage 1 it's important to remember that energy really is finite, and if you do too much you're certain to crash.

Stage 2: Tired and Wired

In stage 2, our mitochondrial energy production may still be low, but our adrenals are working hard to compensate. Adrenal energy feels more 'buzzy' and harder to control and it presents as a feeling of being 'tired and wired.'

Furthermore, when we're on the healing journey and moving from stage 1 to stage 2, our energy tends to go first to our nervous system, and again it's experienced as a tired and wired feeling. This means that although we're making progress it may not feel like it, and some people can even feel as if they're getting worse.

Signs That You're In It

At stage 1 we tend to find that we want to sleep all of the time, and at stage 2, we may find the opposite – we feel tired but we can't sleep. We may notice we feel irritable, more emotionally volatile, and more despondent. At stage 1 we can be too tired to feel our emotions, while at stage 2 they can be quite volatile.

When moving from stage 1 to stage 2, we can also sometimes notice new symptoms – this is a result of our nervous system having more energy. It's a perverse sign of progress, although it hardly feels like it.

How to Move Through It

One of the keys to navigating stage 2 is calming our nervous system and grounding our energy into our body. Firstly, working on calming our nervous system and cultivating a healing state become critical. Because there is some energy in our body, we can manage limited activity at stage 2; however, this must be done extremely carefully and by following the guidelines in the last chapter.

At stage 2, the state we're in when we do things can be very important – we may find that if we keep our system calm, and do things that make us feel good, we can do more activity than we could otherwise.

Stage 3: Reintegration

At stage 3, our energy is increasing again, and we'll find we have more capacity to do things. However, we'll still find that if we do too much, too quickly, we'll crash. If we've previously been somewhat isolated, a particular challenge at stage 3 is reintegrating ourselves into the world. For example, we may have learnt to calm our nervous system and be in a healing state when we're alone and are carefully staying within our energy limits, but find that we're easily triggered outside of this comfort zone when we're around other people or do too much activity.

At stage 3 we can also start to notice that our underlying personality patterns – such as the achiever and helper – resurface, particularly as we reintegrate into society. So working on these again will likely be important.

Signs That You're In It

You'll find that you're able to do more activity – and sometimes you may feel relatively normal – but that doing too much will still result in a crash. You'll likely notice a contrast between how you feel in your comfort zone and how you feel when you're around others. You might feel frustrated as old patterns come back in, and struggle to figure out how to integrate the new person you've become on the healing journey with the person you used to be, so you can function in the world.

How to Move Through It

One of the real keys to moving through stage 3 is working on staying in a healing state when around other people, and integrating the new person you've become into the world. This can often mean creating new boundaries with people, and facing some important decisions about the kind of life you want to live on the other side of your fatigue journey.

At stage 3, the state we're in when we do things becomes critical. Because our body is now well on the road to recovery, a shift in our nervous system can sometimes appear quite miraculous, in terms of how we feel physically.

At this point you might be wondering whether *everyone* goes through these exact recovery stages. The answer is no – this is a model and it's not perfect; however, the vast majority of people do follow some version of this.

Furthermore, not going through all of the recovery stages can have consequences. For example, not going through stage 3 can mean that we keep oscillating between stage 2 and normal functioning because we don't properly learn how to live in a new way in the world. And not going through stage 1 can mean that we get stuck in stage 2 because we've never really slowed down enough to experience the real, deep rest and healing that needs to take place to fuel our journey through stage 2, into stage 3, and eventually full recovery.

Making More Energy Than You're Spending

Identifying the stage of recovery you're at will help determine whether your priority is deep rest (stage 1), calming your nervous system (stage 2), or reintegrating into life while managing your activity carefully and keeping your nervous system calm (stage 3).

However, regardless of which stage you're at, it's absolutely critical that you're making more energy than you're spending. Here's a way to think about this... Let's say you have $100 a day of net income to live on. If your daily expenditure also totals $100 you're able to meet the demand and don't have stress; that is, of course, until you have a day with an unexpected bill. Therefore, prudent financial management would be spending $70 a day and saving the difference to have a reserve, or in energy terms, building up some resilience.

Now, if you're constantly spending $120 a day, you're gradually going into debt. You might get away with this for a while by using credit cards, loans, and overdrafts, but if you don't stop, at some point you're going to go bust. In health terms, that looks like illness.

And to make matters worse, developing fatigue means our income's going down. Let's say our income decreases from $100 a day to $50 a day. Initially, we may attempt to ignore this and not change our lifestyle, but if our expenditure stays at $100 we won't be able to get away with that for very long.

However, there is a pattern I see very often and it goes like this. Someone's living on $100 a day net income but $110 expenditure; gradually they get into debt, otherwise known as getting fatigue. Their income then drops to $80, and they have little choice but to make changes in their life – perhaps they start to work part time or give up some hobbies or social contact. They manage to cut their expenditure from $110 to $90, and at this point they say, 'I've changed my life, so how come I'm still so exhausted?'

Well, if their income's dropped to $80 and their expenditure is still $90, their system is still stressed because the demand exceeds the supply available. This pattern often continues over time as well – the income drops to $50 but the expenditure drops to only $60.

Discover Your Baseline

To put it bluntly, just as with paying off financial debt, healing doesn't start until our income exceeds our expenditure. In fatigue terms, we don't start healing until we're making more energy than we're spending. Without this shift, our body isn't in a healing state because we're using our stress energy to keep going (remember our discussion about the adrenals in Chapter 10?) Healing isn't being prioritized because our body is using all of its resources just to survive.

The more fatigued we become, the fewer resources we have to meet our life, and the more stressed we become by simple things. As we become more stressed, over time we become more fatigued. Until we break this cycle, we're using all of our precious resources just to survive; and whatever else we're doing will fail to work until we redress this imbalance.

Indeed, discovering your 'baseline' – how much activity you should be doing – and learning to pace your activity is so important that it's step 10 of our 12 steps together:

Step 10: Discover your baseline and learn to pace

In fact, I don't think it would be overstating it to say that, more than anything else we've covered in our journey together, getting your activity levels right and discovering which stage of recovery you're at are utterly critical to your healing. Of course, doing so is made all the more challenging by the lack of medical understanding we touched on at the start of the last chapter.

In order to manage your activity levels, you need to discover your baseline – this is the level at which you're able to keep your activity stable and constant. Just as with a bank account, you'll be paying in a little more than you're taking out each day.

Here's the key thing about a baseline – you don't decide a baseline, and you don't 'make it happen.' You *discover* a baseline. A true baseline reveals itself when you slow down and listen to your body. Your baseline is the level at which you're able to maintain your regular activities without your symptoms increasing or your energy becoming more depleted. Returning to our income versus expenditure analogy above, it's the level at which you're paying in more than you're withdrawing in a sustainable way.

Discovering your baseline is significantly easier when you have a certain amount of routine and a predictable and consistent structure to your days and weeks. If you're in a boom-and-bust cycle where one week you do too much and the next week you crash and have to rest to recover from it, you need to stop doing this. To truly stabilize a baseline, you need to stay in line with it fairly consistently, and be able to make predictable and sensible decisions on your activity levels from this place.

Bouncing the Boundaries

Once you have your baseline and it's stable and predictable, and assuming your energy is now returning as a result of addressing the underlying issues we explored in Part II, you can start to increase your activity levels. Our principle for doing this at the OHC is called 'bouncing the boundaries,' and it follows a very specific sequence that we'll come to in a moment.

Bouncing the boundaries means finding your edge and strategically and carefully testing it. You don't force it, and you don't push it – instead, you take a considered step toward increasing your activity. For example, if you've been reliably walking for 10 minutes a day at baseline, one day you might try walking for 11 minutes. Or, if you've been reliably walking for 45 minutes a day, you might try walking much faster for one of these minutes.

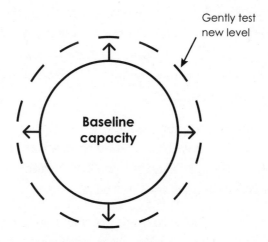

Bouncing the boundaries

However, one of the golden rules of bouncing the boundaries, particularly in the early stages of the healing journey, is that initially, you don't maintain that increase in your activity levels. If you've gone from 10 minutes to 11 minutes, you then go back to 10 minutes for a few days, to be sure.

Remember the delayed fatigue response we talked about in Chapter 3? Well, the reason we're being cautious is that we know the impact of that increase may not be felt immediately. Indeed, when bouncing the boundaries, we need to be careful not to stack multiple bounces in a row because sometimes the effect can be cumulative.

How to Bounce the Boundaries

In summary, the steps to go through when bouncing the boundaries are as follows:

1. Find your baseline – this is the level at which your energy and your symptoms are stable. You should be building a little more energy than you're spending each day.

2. If you feel that you have a little more energy, or want to test the baseline you're at, test by gently increasing your level of activity. This will usually be in the range of a 5–10 percent increase, but in more sensitive instances it might be a 1–2 percent change.

3. Do this increase only *once* and then return to baseline for, say, 3 days. If you experience no ill effects, try this increase again, but with a shorter gap in between. So, rather than waiting 2–3 days, try 1 or 2 days.

4. Once you can comfortably maintain this new level of activity, consider it your new baseline. After a short period to stabilize it, you can explore the next level. However, bear in mind that some activities may only be possible with enough recovery time afterward.

5. If at any point you have a flare-up of your symptoms, return to your previous baseline and consolidate again there. You

may also find you need to drop to your previous baseline temporarily, to rebuild back to this baseline.

———————

I appreciate that being so careful with your activity levels can feel like being locked in a prison. And if you're at the milder end of the fatigue spectrum this might also seem rather overdramatic, so you can have a much lighter touch when integrating these principles. However, I've dedicated a full chapter to these ideas because for many people they really are a critical part of the foundation of their healing.

No amount of good nutrition, calming your nervous system, or addressing underlying imbalances, such as those we've been exploring, will help you circumnavigate the fact that for your body to recover, it has to do so in a stable and careful way. If you have the discipline and patience to bear with this approach, the rewards can be life transforming.

Let's return to James's story, with which we opened this chapter. After a year or so of using the approach to activity outlined in this chapter, alongside being fully committed to the rest of his OHC plan, James made a full recovery.

James knew this had happened when he found himself cycling almost 200 miles (320 km) in two days, without experiencing any negative consequences. And he knew he was going to be OK doing this because he was still listening to his body every step of the way.

Here's how I believe you have to think about it: you're not retreating because you're defeated; you're retreating in order to build the substance and foundation for a sustainable, and ultimately effective, attack.

However, it's not only down to managing our activity levels. We have a somewhat famous phrase at the OHC: 'It's not just what you do – it's the state you're in when you do it.' Sometimes we can do the same activity on two different days, in two different states, and it'll have an entirely different effect. In the next chapter we're going to explore how you can transform your state, something that has the potential to directly impact your energy levels.

■■ Chapter 15 ■■

CULTIVATING A HEALING STATE

In Chapter 8 we looked at Colin's story and the seemingly miraculous transformation that occurred when he acted 'as if' there was nothing wrong and got his body into a deep healing state. This had such an impact on me that understanding how to calm the nervous system and cultivate a healing state became a key focus for many years.

For some people, cultivating a healing state can appear to be as simple as flicking off a switch. For others, it can be much more complex and involve multiple layers of therapeutic work, including healing underlying traumas that are held in the body.

The situation is also significantly complicated by the uncertainty of suffering from a medically unexplained illness, the fluctuating nature of fatigue, and the constant lack of understanding from those around us. As we've discussed, the net result of all this is that we can end up in the exact opposite state to the one we need to be in to heal.

In this chapter, we're going to explore some fundamental principles that'll help calm your system – with a particular focus on simple exercises you can get started on right away.

The Power of Mindfulness

Meditation is perhaps the most talked-about tool in personal development and alternative healing. The claims for its benefits can at times sound far-fetched, and if you're anything like I was when I started, they can also feel a very long way from where you're at now.

When I began meditating back in 1998, as a tool to support my healing journey, the picture was very different to how it is today. At that time, meditation teachings were more likely to be found in a backstreet New Age crystal shop than in the mainstream media, where they are available now.

Although forms of meditation and prayer are used in different religions and can have certain connotations, the form of meditation that I teach is separate from any spiritual or religious practice. My focus is simply toward calming the mind, coming into the body, and connecting into the present moment.

What we're looking to cultivate in meditation is *mindfulness*, which can be defined as: 'A mental state achieved by focusing one's awareness on the present moment, while calmly acknowledging and accepting one's feelings, thoughts, and bodily sensations, used as a therapeutic technique.'

When we calm and relax our mind and body, and connect into the present moment, we're directly encouraging our body into a healing state.

Changing Your Brainwaves

The calmer your nervous system becomes and the more deeply connected you are to the present moment, the more easily you can listen to your body and its communications. You see, to listen to your body, you have to actually *be* in it (as opposed to being lost in your thinking mind in your head), which is what meditation allows you to do. However, beyond its impact on your body, meditation has a very real effect on the function of your brain.

The Four Brainwave Patterns

Research has shown that we have four categories of brainwave patterns. All are present all of the time, but different brainwaves are dominant in different situations, depending on which state we're in.

1. **Beta** is a state of concentrated thought and higher mental arousal. When we're working our brain hard, and/or are overstimulated or stressed, we have an excess of beta.

2. **Alpha** is a state of relaxed thought and gentle mental arousal. When we're relaxed, living in the moment and in a healing state, we have a dominance of alpha.

3. **Theta** is daydreaming and dreaming sleep. When we have an excess of theta at night, we'll tend to feel irritable and unrefreshed. Our nervous system doesn't distinguish between something that's real and something that's vividly imagined, so when we dream we're being chased by a saber-toothed tiger, it feels real to our nervous system.

4. **Delta** is a state of deep sleep, and it's in deep sleep that our body heals and restores itself, releasing things such as growth hormone. There is a direct correlation between the amount of delta sleep we get and how refreshed we feel in the morning.

When we're in a stress state, we tend to have an excess of beta during the day and a lack of alpha. That means our system isn't just working harder, it's also lacking time to restore and regenerate.

One of the functions of theta, or dreaming sleep, is to process and organize the thoughts we have during the day. So, the more beta we have during the day, the more theta we tend to have at night, which ultimately means we have more tiring dreaming sleep and less healing deep sleep.

Furthermore, for deep sleep to happen, we have to relax fully and let go. Just like a caveman living in fear of the saber-toothed tiger that's been hunting him, in a stress state we sleep with one eye half open, not fully surrendering to the peace and quiet within.

So, beyond everything we've already explored in Chapter 8 about the importance of being in a healing state, the more we calm our mind, the more of a direct impact we have on how much energy we consume during the day, and how much we reset and restore at night.

Although there are a number of techniques we might need to reset our nervous system, for many people meditation is a critical foundation. When you calm your beta and increase your alpha during the day, you have less mental tiredness and deeper rest.

The calmer your mind is during the day, the more deep sleep you'll get when you rest at night. Indeed, when it comes to working with patients with sleep issues, my primary focus is always to calm their mind and nervous system during the day. If we're calmer during the day, our sleep will more naturally take care of itself.

Four Types of Meditation

Learning to meditate can feel rather overwhelming – where do we even start, with so many different practices and schools of thought? When it comes to the various types of meditation, I'd argue that they aren't all equal in their value of helping you cultivate a healing state, although they do each have their benefits.[155–157] It's far from a complete list, but I tend to categorize them into the following four types.

1: State-Changing Practices

These are practices designed to cultivate a change in our state, often to activate an experience of bliss or euphoria. This includes mantra-based practices such as transcendental meditation and energy-focused practices such as kundalini.

2: Intention-Based and Visualization Practices

These are designed to focus the mind toward a particular thing, such as a relaxing beach or a calming forest. The idea is that by taking the mind there, the body will respond as though it's really there (remember what I said about the nervous system not distinguishing between something that's real and something that's vividly imagined?)

3: Hypnosis and Suggestion Practices

These are designed to focus the mind on certain ideas and principles that'll encourage a particular outcome.

4: Body-Based Meditation Practices

These use the body as a focus of meditation, encouraging us to relax and feel more fully into it. My experience with patients is that body-based meditation practices tend to be the most helpful for those with fatigue, for a few reasons. Firstly, the more fully we relax into and feel our body, the better we get at actually listening to it. Secondly, we tend to become more grounded and connected to the present moment with body-based practices than we do with other, more stimulating, practices.[156, 158, 159]

Finally, by actively learning to let go of our thoughts and come more into the body and the present moment, we're able to continue our practice outside of our formal meditation sessions – in our daily life – whereas other practices may require us to listen to recordings. So,

I'm not saying that you shouldn't explore other practices or that you won't receive any benefit from them, but my suggestion would be at the very least to incorporate some body-based meditation practices into your day.

How Do You Meditate?

The practice of meditation is remarkably simple, but it's not easy. Really what we're learning to do is let go of our focus on any particular thoughts or paths of thinking and connect into the present moment. When thoughts come into our mind we're observing them, letting them go, and shifting our focus to our body.

My first meditation teacher would say that thoughts are trains and the mind is a train station through which the thoughts (trains) pass – you observe each train (thought) but you don't board it, you just watch it pass you by. It was a logical metaphor, but one that left me feeling more overwhelmed.

You see, he was talking about our local provincial train station in Southeast England, which had a few trains an hour, whereas my mind felt more like New York's Grand Central Terminal or London King's Cross, with multiple trains leaving at any one time. I used to wonder which was the train I was supposed to be observing but not boarding, when there were so many in any given moment!

What I find more helpful is teaching my patients and students to do their best to observe their thoughts and let them go, but ultimately to feel into and connect to the sensations of their body. Focusing on the breath can be a helpful part of this, although for some people this can become a source of stress in itself; if this is the case I just have people feel into and connect to the sensation of their arms and legs, where there tends to be less emotional material stored.

With regard to the many details related to meditation – including how long to practice for and at what time of day, how you should sit, how you should breathe – my feeling is that although these can be relevant in some situations, the most important thing is to get started with a practice you can stick with. A consistent 10 minutes a day, at a time that works for you, is always better than an occasional session at 6 a.m. that leaves you wiped out for the rest of the day.

The problem with writing and talking about meditation is that it can only do so much in helping us to actually practice meditation. So I've recorded a guided meditation for you in the style I'm describing above, and it's waiting for you as part of the companion course. You can download the meditation from there and use it as often as you like: www.alexhoward.com/fatigue.

Resetting the Homeostatic Balance

Meditation is enormously helpful, and for many people it's a key tool in their toolbox for helping cultivate a healing state; however, like any practice it does have its limitations, and on its own it's rarely enough. One of the limitations is that even if we've been successful in calming and relaxing our system, between each meditation practice the body gradually becomes stimulated into a stress state once more.

When we don't understand why this is happening, it can be enormously frustrating. We work hard to calm and relax the system, and almost the moment we stop it seems to begin to rewire itself immediately. This is because the body has normalized being in a state of stress and it's simply returning to what it believes to be its point of balance.

The body has all kinds of 'homeostatic' balances, which it needs to carefully manage and maintain at any point in time. From our blood pressure, blood sugar, and body temperature, to our metabolism, heart rate, and circadian rhythms, our body normalizes and works hard to maintain whatever balances we become used to. If we're living in a state of maladaptive stress response, our body doesn't return to this state by accident – it does it because it believes that is where balance lies.

To retrain this balance, we have to first build more awareness of what's happening in our nervous system and what's triggering it. The more we notice those moments when our system attempts to return to its maladaptive balance, the more we're empowered to shift our focus and reset our system.

In Chapter 6 we explored the five energy depleting personality patterns of the achiever, helper, anxiety, perfectionist, and controller. Well, along with happening on a macro behavioral level, these also play out moment to moment in our thinking and behaviors.

For example, let's say you're resting on the sofa at the end of the day. Your body is clearly communicating that it's tired but your mind is saying, *I need to go and finish that project for work.* And in the next breath it says, *I didn't return Katie's call, like I promised, and she needs my support.* And then a few seconds later you start to worry about how you'll feel in the morning and what symptoms you might have on the way into work.

In this example, your body is being very clear about its need for rest; however, your mind has just run an achiever pattern (the work project), helper pattern (worrying about Katie), and anxiety pattern (about your symptoms the next day). Do these patterns encourage a state of healing for your body, or do they serve to activate your nervous system? You got it – these thoughts are actively triggering the body into a state of agitation, exactly at the time it should be resting.

To help you better identify these patterns as they're playing out, here's a checklist you can run through.

Personality Patterns Checklist

Achiever

- Are you pushing your body to do things it doesn't really have the energy to do?

- Are you overcommitting to projects in an attempt to achieve a sense of self-worth?

- Do you resist rest in a bid to stay busy?

Helper

- Do you find yourself ignoring your body's needs and putting others first?

- Do other people's needs feel more important than your own?

- Do you ask others for help, or do you find that you're always the one being asked?

Anxiety

- Is your mind always racing with thoughts?

- Do you find yourself constantly analyzing situations, and trying to work out what to do?

- Do you experience feelings of mental confusion and overwhelm, with your mind racing?

Perfectionist

- Does getting things right feel hugely important to you?

- Do you agonize over details that others would let go?

- Do you get caught in a form of paralysis and overwhelm while trying to get things right?

Controller

- Do things need to be done in a certain way for you to feel safe?

- Do you attempt to control others' actions to allow yourself to feel better?

- Do you find yourself avoiding situations where you can't control the environment?

My point here is not that you need to become the thought police of every thought you might ever have, or that you somehow need to learn to 'control your mind.' Indeed, neither of those things will ultimately work. However, we do need to learn to catch such patterns and come to gradually retrain our mental habits.

Rewiring Your Brain

One of the areas I found most fascinating when studying for my psychology degree was how the human brain works. Even today, with all the technical wizardry we can do with computers, we can't come close to some of the masterful potentials of the brain.

I was particularly interested in the impact of neural plasticity, which is the process by which the brain learns and retains habits and behaviors. For example, when we have a particular pattern of thinking a number of times, our brain then learns to do this automatically – we literally wire a pattern of learning in our brain. The more we think this thought pattern, the stronger the neural pathway becomes.

If after many years of running a particular thought pattern we want to change it, we're at first fighting against well-established neural pathways. Let's say you've been driving home from work along the same route for many years and then one day you move to a new home and your route changes. You've become so conditioned to driving the old route that, if you don't concentrate hard, you may find yourself driving to your old house.

Two Steps for Changing Your Thought Patterns

Although learning to change these patterns can be a significant focus in itself – indeed, it's a key part of my online coaching program, the RESET Program – there are a couple of top tips I want to leave you with now.

Step 1: Awareness

If you can see it, you don't have to be it. The more clearly you can see and catch these patterns, the more empowered you are to change them. It takes time and it takes practice, but it's absolutely possible, and the only place you can start is where you are now.

Step 2: Discipline and Diligence

You're actively retraining your brain and creating new neural pathways, but you need to be diligent and consistent until your brain learns a new way of functioning. Each time you catch yourself and move in a different direction, you're actively rewiring your brain.

Let's return to the example from a little earlier, in which your mind's running an achiever pattern about pushing through to finish a work project when your body needs rest. Being aware that this is your achiever pattern playing out gives you a choice you didn't have before.

In the past, you'd likely have been a slave to the pattern and ignored your body, but by having awareness, you can make a different choice – to listen to it instead. This might look like having a long soak in the bath to relax your body, going to bed early, or taking a long hard look at your schedule for the coming few days to see if you can give yourself some time out.

By catching the old pattern, making a better choice, and having the discipline to follow through with it, you're taking an important step toward cultivating a new habit and pattern. And if your body feels better for it, that'll only further reinforce the new direction of listening to and nurturing it.

Now that we've looked at some of the core psychology principles of fatigue, in the next chapter we're going to start exploring some of the key nutrition principles. We're going to see how we can optimize the fuel you give your mitochondria.

■■ Chapter 16 ■■

NUTRITION FUNDAMENTALS

O ne of the decisions I made on the back of that life-changing conversation with my uncle, two years into my chronic fatigue journey, was to become a vegetarian. Having read various books on the merits of a vegetarian lifestyle for both our own health and that of the planet, I was strongly persuaded.

It wasn't an easy change for me. Growing up, I was a fussy eater and would eat only two vegetables: peas and potatoes. Despite some determined efforts by family members to expand my repertoire, I was stubborn to the point where I'd sit at the table for hours on end, refusing to eat. Short of force-feeding me, they had little choice but to accept my self-imposed limits. My grandmother did her best to circumnavigate these by regularly making fresh soup, which for some reason I was quite happy to eat, as long as it was sieved!

After becoming a vegetarian I quickly had to expand my repertoire of foods, but when it came down to it, that was a small price to pay for a potential improvement in my health. I continued with the vegetarian diet for four years; however, unfortunately, despite my willingness, there was no discernable change. I finally realized why when I attended a workshop by the health writer Leslie Kenton.

Leslie Kenton had been one of the foremost figures in the raw food movement, which promoted the importance of eating raw food and avoiding all sources of animal protein. As an early version of the current focus on a plant-based diet, her raw food principles had made total sense, but the reality for me had been less positive.

Kenton's now directly opposite argument about the benefits, and for many people the necessity, of animal protein for cultivating health, was compelling. Apart from presenting some powerful research, more importantly to me, Leslie had the testimony of her own health transformation. In particular, she emphasized the impact of animal protein on balancing blood sugar levels and supporting adrenal health. At this point I was close to full recovery, although blood sugar and adrenal fatigue was still something I struggled with. I was constantly hungry and I never felt fully satisfied by my meals.

Having become used to running experiments on my body and testing any new hypothesis, whether I agreed with it or not, I decided to try eating animal protein daily for a week. The effect was staggering. My energy levels increased, as did the stability of my energy. In fact, within a month I took my final step back to full recovery and returning to normal exercise levels.

A year later, I met nutritional therapist Niki Gratrix, who you'll remember from her exuberant discovery of the importance of our mitochondria. Niki had spent the last two years transitioning to a raw food diet and would regularly drink only freshly made vegetable juice for days on end. Our diets could not have been more opposite and we had many 'spirited debates' about who was right. For months, Niki and I presented each other with research studies, case studies of people we'd worked with, and anything else we could lay our hands on to win the running debate.

In the end, we realized the only way to break the status quo was to run another experiment. I wasn't willing to give up meat, but I was open to adding freshly squeezed green vegetable juices to my diet at least once a day. Niki wasn't willing to give up her focus on raw food, but she was willing to try eating some organic meat. The result? My energy levels went up again, and Niki's energy levels became more stable. Niki's body didn't seem to need anything like as much meat as mine did to have the same effect, but she couldn't deny the benefit.

Why a Balanced Diet Matters

At this point you might be wondering why I've taken several pages to share the intricate details of my dietary history. Well, I've done so to make a critical point about food – albeit one that's rather inconvenient: biochemically, we're all different.

In fact, as the OHC has continued to flourish over the years and we've worked with so many people, I can tell you with great confidence that my opinion on this has only become stronger. When it comes to food, one person's medicine really is another person's poison.

I say that this point is inconvenient because in a book such as this I'm supposed to tell you which diet plan to follow to help increase your energy, and I'm afraid I can't do that. The truth is that I've no idea how your body will respond to different foods, and once again, the point I've labored throughout this book still stands – you need to learn to listen to your own body, regardless of what anyone else says. What I can do though is give you some orienting principles to help direct you, and I can certainly give you guidance on certain foods to avoid and why.

Although of course not everyone with fatigue has a bad diet, many of us have got used to eating in a way that's not just suboptimal, it's also having a direct effect on our energy levels. As we discussed in Chapter 10, when we explored your hormones, it's also the case that when your energy's low, you're more likely to choose stimulants to keep you going.

The classically 'bad' Western diet is very high in processed foods such as pasta, white bread, potato chips, cakes, cookies, sweets (candy), sodas, and fizzy drinks. A diet high in these foods, which are called refined carbohydrates, is often by default low in other important elements such as fiber, protein, good fats, vitamins, and minerals.

Achieving a good balance within our diet, and also ensuring that the right ratio of foods are present on the plate, is critical to everything else we've discussed in this book. Indeed, through the lens of what we've covered so far, we want to eat food to help:

- Provide the crucial nutrients to fuel our mitochondria to make energy

- Maintain blood sugar (glucose) and associated energy balance (more on this below), which is important to help reduce the load on our maladaptive stress response and hormone function

- Support our overall digestive function and gut microbiome, which includes avoiding food intolerances (more on this below) and taking the overall load off our digestive system

- Provide nutrients to support hormone balance, including our adrenal function

- Provide nutrients to support immune function and our body's detoxification processes

As you can see, what you eat is about so much more than just being healthy – it has a direct impact on almost everything we've looked at together in this book. Indeed, what you eat is so important that it's our eleventh step together:

Step 11: Optimize your food

Although there are many factors we could explore with regard to what you eat, beyond what we explored in Chapter 9, I want to emphasize two other principles – your blood sugar and food intolerances.

The Blood Glucose Roller Coaster

One way to think about your blood glucose, or blood sugar, is as a source of energy for your body. Although this is an oversimplification, we want to have a stable blood sugar level to provide us with consistent energy. Blood sugar levels that are too high are a sign of diabetes, and too low is hypoglycemia, which causes our adrenals to work hard to bring things back into balance.

If our diet is dominated by refined carbohydrates such as bread and white rice and isn't balanced by an intake of fiber, protein, and complex carbohydrates such as whole grains and vegetables, it will drive our insulin levels too high, which will ultimately negatively impact our blood glucose management. At the OHC, we refer to this as 'the blood glucose roller coaster' (see diagram below).

Put simply, leaving too long a gap between meals or eating only foods that are absorbed too quickly, such as refined carbohydrates, will cause a spike in our blood sugar levels, followed by a crash. During the crash, we reach for more quickly absorbed foods, such as chocolate, to stabilize ourselves, and the cycle is repeated.

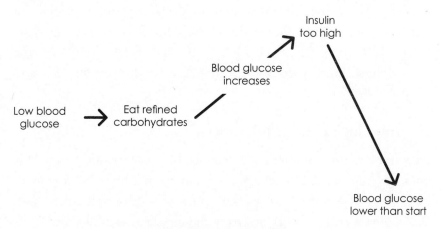

The blood glucose roller coaster

The Impact of the Blood Glucose Roller Coaster

As I mentioned in Chapter 10, this cycle can cause an array of symptoms, including:

- Sugar cravings

- Excess sweating

- Dizziness

- Fatigue

- Blurred vision

- Trembling or shakiness

- A fast pulse or palpitations

- Irritability

- Difficulty concentrating and confusion

One of the likely impacts of this cycle is a release of stress hormones, which triggers the maladaptive stress response and further perpetuates the cycle. The good news is that it's usually relatively simple to stabilize our blood sugar. How do we do it? Well, we need to eat a healthy balance of protein, fats, and carbohydrates, specifically avoiding eating carbohydrates on their own. We'll come back to this shortly.

Do You Have Food Intolerances?

Do you ever find that after eating you feel significantly more tired? Or perhaps symptoms such as bloating or brain fog are worsened? You might even find this seems to happen with certain foods in particular. Well, this could be a direct result of what's known as a food intolerance.[160, 161]

Food intolerance is where our immune system reacts to a food as though it might be a danger to us. (Please note that this is very different to a food allergy, where people can have an immediate and sometimes life-threatening reaction to eating certain foods.)

Research demonstrates that the inflammation and immune activation caused by food intolerances may directly affect our mitochondria, and therefore our energy production.[71, 106, 161] Food intolerances can also create a number of other symptoms, including:

- Burping and bloating

- Headaches and brain fog

- Indigestion

- Nasal congestion

- Musculoskeletal pain

In fact, sometimes the worst reactions to foods aren't digestive symptoms – they're the dreaded symptoms of a foggy brain or a headache. Although there are many different foods we can have an intolerance to,[162] many of us have issues with dairy and gluten. We'll come back to this later.

The Dos and Don'ts of Digestion

Now that we've looked at the importance of managing your blood sugar, and the potential impact of food intolerances, let's explore some general dos and don'ts that'll help you address both of these issues, along with the potential underlying digestive issues we explored in Chapter 9.

Dietary Dos

Eat Protein

Include a source of protein with each meal and snack. Protein may help to slow the release of glucose and can therefore help to balance blood sugar levels,[163] as well as provide building blocks for hormones and muscles. Good sources of protein include eggs, fish, poultry, plain live yogurt, goats' cheese, tempeh (tofu), nuts, seeds, pulses, legumes, red meat, and protein powders. A helpful way to think about this is to ensure that at least 30 percent of any plate of food is made up of protein-rich foods.

Choose Good Fats

Fat has suffered from all kinds of image problems over the years. However, it's important to make a distinction between good (unsaturated) fats such as olive oil or nut oils and bad (saturated) fats such as butter or cheese. A small amount of good fat is critical to health and needed as a source of essential fatty acids, which our body cannot make itself. Essential fatty acids are important for a number of things, including hormone function.[164] Fats also help with the absorption of various vitamins, including Vitamin A, Vitamin D, and Vitamin E.

Sources of good fat include oily fish such as salmon, mackerel, sardines, and rainbow trout. When selecting fish, your order of preference should be as follows: freshly caught, frozen, smoked, in a glass jar, and then canned. Other sources include nuts and seeds such as almonds, cashews, walnuts, Brazil nuts, sunflower, flax, and chia seeds; also avocados and olive oil (preferably extra virgin).

Eat a Rainbow

Make your plate as colorful as possible by choosing a variety of vegetables and salad – this ensures you're getting a wide range of vitamins and minerals in your diet.[165] Aim to fill at least half your plate with different vegetables, ideally at every meal, including breakfast. This is easily achieved by having a vegetable omelet at breakfast or thinking outside the box and considering vegetable soup or a green smoothie containing spinach or kale.

Aim to have 6–8 portions of vegetables per day, and no more than two portions of fruit (due to its high sugar content). By eating a wide range of vegetables, you'll also be ensuring your body gets enough fiber, which, among other things, is important for healthy bowel function and supporting a healthy balance of gut bacteria.[166–168]

Time Your Meals and Eat Regularly

When your body's healthy and balanced you should aim to eat every 3–5 hours, and within an hour of getting up in the morning.[169] Sometimes, to keep blood sugar levels balanced, you may need to eat more or less often than this, so as always, listen to your body. A subgroup of people (myself included) find that a modest snack before bed can significantly improve the quality of their sleep.

Although there is growing evidence of the value of intermittent fasting (going for extended periods in the day without food),[170, 171] those with sensitive adrenals can find this detrimental. Remember, as always, your body knows best when it comes to deciding how often you need to eat, and you need to listen to it.

Switch to Organic

An organic diet is ideal for minimizing exposure to antibiotics, pesticides, fertilizers, and other chemicals, and increasing levels of some nutrients.[172] Some organic foods can be costlier than non-organic ones, and organic foods may not always be available, so simply do the best you can. If you can't afford to eat a 100 percent organic diet, prioritize sourcing organic meat, dairy, and eggs. Game tends to be organic and it can be reasonably priced. Free-range or grass-fed is the next best choice. Always wash and peel your plant foods to at least reduce your exposure to pesticides.

Stay Hydrated

Ideally you should consume around 4 pints (2 liters) of fluid a day.[173] This includes fluid from your food, so the amount you need to drink is about 2–3 pints (1–1.5 liters). Fruit or herbal teas count as fluid, and it's good to drink some plain water each day too. Be aware that fruit juices are high in sugar, so drink them only occasionally and always dilute them 50/50 with water.

Eat Mindfully

As we discussed in Chapter 9, eating in a stressful state has all kinds of impacts on our digestion. We'll likely not chew our food properly, our body's resources will be diverted to functions other than digestion, and we'll also likely undereat or overeat.[174] To eat in a way that supports our body, we need to be connected and listening to it. Some helpful principles are avoiding eating on the go or in front of the television (and if you do, make sure you're doing so slowly and listening to your body), or while you're distracted doing other things.

Dietary Don'ts

Sugar

Avoid refined sugar, white refined carbohydrates, and foods containing sugar such as alcohol, dried fruit, and 100 percent fruit juice. Examples of white refined carbohydrates are white bread, white pasta, cakes, and biscuits. Remember, refined carbohydrates provide a source of energy that's very short-lived and can often be followed by a dip in energy, placing a further strain on your body. Wholegrain, unrefined carbohydrates release their energy more steadily, helping you to maintain more consistent energy levels after your meals.[175]

Gluten and Dairy

I highly recommend that you trial a gluten- and dairy-free diet if possible, as for many people this can make a huge difference – not only to their digestive symptoms but to other symptoms too.[103, 160, 176–179] The ideal would be to start with three months off dairy and six weeks off gluten. However, many people will see improvements in just a few days or weeks.

When eliminating any food, it's normally important to ensure that you don't reduce the volume of food you're eating and that you fill the gap with healthy alternatives. Furthermore, it's also important to replace the foods you remove with foods rich in the same nutrients. For example, when avoiding dairy, you can increase your intake of calcium-rich foods such as cooked spinach, broccoli, peas, beans, almonds, and so on. In the case of a gluten-free diet, ensure you eat good sources of fiber, such as vegetables, and if you can tolerate them, rice, gluten-free quinoa, pulses, and seeds.

Caffeine

Caffeine is a stimulant, and as we discussed in Chapter 10, these are the last things our body needs.[180–183] Caffeine isn't only present in coffee – it's also in tea, cola drinks, cocoa, and in 'energy drinks.' Decaffeinated coffee still contains some caffeine (typically 5 percent) and producers may have used aggressive chemicals and toxic metals in the decaffeination process. Herbal teas such as redbush (also known as rooibos), peppermint, ginger, and chamomile can be useful to drink, and many people are amazed at how their tastes change with time.

Commercially Processed and Convenience Foods

When buying pre-packaged food, check the labels and avoid those containing sweeteners, preservatives, colorings, and words you don't recognize. Usually, the fewer ingredients listed on a label, the better. Processed foods tend to contain added sugar and other sweeteners, which will affect your blood sugar balance.

Other hidden ingredients in processed foods include hydrogenated fats, which can contribute to inflammatory reactions and even heart disease. A general philosophy is that if a food has ingredients that are numbers rather than words, or words you can't pronounce, they're likely not a good source of energy for you!

Eating the Same Foods Every Day

A tempting pattern to get into if you're sensitive to foods and don't particularly enjoy cooking, is eating the same meals day after day. The problem is that, over time, this can create more food sensitivities and also lead to less diversity in the bacteria in your gut microbiome. So, even if you're just varying the vegetables you have, and cycling through a few simple protein sources and carbohydrates, the more diversity in your diet, the better.

The 80/20 Rule

At this point, you'd be forgiven for feeling a little overwhelmed by all we've talked about in this chapter. But here's the thing – you don't need to do all of this perfectly. In fact, any attempt to do so may well end up making things worse, not better.

The goal here is not to fear food – it's to change your relationship with it in such a way that it becomes an optimum energy source to your body. In many cases, if you can follow these principles for 80 percent of the time you'll see enormous benefits, and slipping up for 20 percent of the time is unlikely to cause major problems.

There is just one exception: to truly discover whether you'd benefit from removing gluten or dairy from your diet, you do need to be

100 percent strict for that initial period (three months for dairy, six weeks for gluten).

Having said all this, I'm still aware that we've focused very much on theory here rather than practice. As we touched on earlier, although I certainly can't tell you the perfect diet for you, there are some plans that integrate what we've explored in this chapter and these can be used as a guide. You'll find recipe plans in the companion course at www.alexhoward.com/fatigue.

So, we've explored some practical steps in listening to your body and calming your nervous system, as well as basic nutrition principles, and we now need to turn our attention to working with practitioners. It can be a tricky process, but armed with a few key principles, you can navigate it so much more easily.

■■ Chapter 17 ■■

WORKING WITH PRACTITIONERS

There wasn't one single moment when I made the decision to start The Optimum Health Clinic. As with many things in life, there were lots of small moments over many years that culminated in a decision that felt like it'd made itself. In many ways I was honoring a commitment I'd made to myself to do something to help others in the same horrendous situation in which I'd found myself.

However, I do remember one of those moments very clearly. It was a few months before I decided on the name of the clinic and registered the website domain. I was working another late night in the bedsit where I lived and found myself thinking about all the practitioners I'd consulted over the years on my own journey to healing.

As I sat at my desk, I calculated that I'd seen 36 practitioners; some I'd visited only once, others many times. Each appointment had been its own investment of hope and financial resources; indeed, I'd spent almost my entire student loan on supplements in an attempt to facilitate my healing. Some of these consultations had been worthwhile, others had not; however, all had taught me something valuable about what makes a great clinic – through an example of what to do, or what not to do.

As I thought about the kind of organization I'd dreamed of creating, it wasn't just the obvious things like clinical excellence and being at the forefront of ideas and innovation that were crucial to me. There was also something particularly important about that feeling of being truly seen and understood by the person working with me. When I felt someone was going through the motions, I knew there was a far poorer chance that they'd be able to really decode what was going on in my unique situation.

As we discussed in Chapter 12, you have to be captain of the ship of your own recovery, and you have to be inspired toward the potential we all have to heal. But that clearly doesn't negate the importance of the role of the practitioner; and the relationship between you and any practitioners you're working with is critical.

Choosing a Practitioner

It's my vision that this book will deeply empower you to play an active role in your healing path, and there is so much you can do for yourself – from learning to listen to your body to calming your nervous system and transforming your diet. Although this can all take you a long way, because of the complex nature of fatigue, the chances are that you'll also need input from specialist practitioners.

I do, of course, hope you might choose to work with the practitioner team at The Optimal Health Clinic; indeed, I believe we do a remarkable job of supporting our patients (who live in more than 50 different countries), with more than half of our practitioner team having themselves recovered from fatigue in its many forms.

However, you may find a different path that you feel is a better fit for you, and so in this chapter I want to share certain key principles that'll help you choose a practitioner, prepare for consultations, and get the most out of them. I believe that mastering these skills alone can save you endless heartache and a great deal of money. In fact, this is so important that it's our twelfth and final step together!

Step 12 – Manage your team

At a time in our lives when we feel perhaps at our least resourceful, we can find ourselves thrust into making complex choices about which path to take, who to work with, and how to navigate the healing journey. Sometimes we can also feel like we have to fight to be heard by those who seem to place too much trust in the limits of science, and not enough in the critical information that our body is giving us every day.

Practitioner Red Flags

Although I can't tell you who you should trust or work with, I can tell you what to look out for in any practitioner, be they orthodox medical or from the fields of integrative or alternative medicine. All fields have their visionaries and geniuses, and all have their charlatans and incompetent practitioners. As a starting point, the following is a checklist of red flags I'd look out for in a practitioner:

Doesn't Have Specialist Experience

Fatigue is a complex condition with its own unique characteristics. To really understand its many nuances a practitioner needs to be seeing more than a few people a year. After all, if someone's suffering with a heart condition, they're referred to a cardiologist not a general practitioner. If you're working with a generalist practitioner, you may well find you know more than they do about the nuances of your condition.

Claims to Have All the Answers

As much as we might wish it to be so, no one has a 100 percent success rate. As soon as someone uses phrases such as 'I can cure you,' or 'I can guarantee you'll recover with this approach,' you shouldn't wait around to hear another word. Such claims are usually an example of one of two things – the practitioner is either lying outright and knows full well they don't have such success, or perhaps even worse, they're suffering from a severe case of confirmation bias, which we'll discuss in a while.

Makes You Feel as if It's All Your Fault

When a particular approach doesn't work, we usually place the blame on one of three things: the methodology, the practitioner's application of it, or our ability to put our part into action. Personally, I'm of the opinion that if someone works with me and they walk away with things having failed to progress, and believe that they're to blame for it, they're worse off than they were at the start. They not only still have the same set of issues but they also have the burden of believing that they're to blame.

When methodologies aren't the right fit for someone, practitioners can be very quick to pass the responsibility from themselves and the approach they're using onto the client. For me, this in itself is a red flag. I'm not suggesting that the active participation of the patient isn't critical (it very much is – remember what we discussed in chapters 1 and 12), it's just that it's far too easy to blame the patient rather than go digging for the limitations in an approach or the practitioner's application of it. At the OHC our protocol has been shaped more by the lessons of those we've *not* helped in the way we would hope, than those we have.

Is Disrespectful of Other Practitioners

A certain amount of professional rivalry is inevitable, and it's also healthy because it drives practitioners to be better. However, when this moves from a passion for a particular approach and its merits to speaking in a derogatory way about other approaches and practitioners, I think that again, we should be concerned. Indeed, my experience is that everyone has different pieces of the truth, and just because someone sees something differently to me, that doesn't make either of us right or wrong. Curious and truth-seeking practitioners will place a higher value on learning and getting better at their craft than always being right and putting others down. Professional discernment is healthy, but being disrespectful of the work of others is not.

Uses Fear Tactics to Motivate You to Take Action

The last thing anyone suffering from fatigue needs is to have their fears and anxieties used for someone else's gain. I think the way that the internet has democratized health is a great thing, but when I see articles headlined 'The 5 things you must know to avoid illness,' or 'If you don't follow this program your fatigue will get worse,' I immediately lose respect for the author. Even if the information they're sharing is valid, framing it in such a way is playing to people's fears, and that's the opposite of what they need.

Beyond these red flags, there is another fundamental issue to look out for in practitioners – confirmation bias.

The Danger of Confirmation Bias

Confirmation bias is a phrase more commonly used to understand political views – we hold a certain belief or perspective and we interpret evidence in such a way that reinforces those views. If someone presents evidence that supports our views, we're open to it – we talk about it to others and we use it to confirm our already held ideas. However, if someone presents information that contradicts our views, we treat it differently. Perhaps we ignore it or minimize its significance. Or perhaps we look for flaws in it, or question its source, and generally defend against even the clear logic in front of us.

Part of what's fascinating about confirmation bias is that it goes beyond the way we treat information. We also tend to surround ourselves with people who support our views. In fact, we virtually curate our relationships to deepen our immersion in the bubble in which we live. Technology will also help us along the way. Indeed, the algorithms of social platforms such as Facebook and Instagram will learn through our behaviors what we do and don't believe to be true, and will serve up information that further supports our perspective to make us feel comfortable and spend more time on the platform (allowing them to make more advertising revenue).

How does this apply to health, you might be wondering. Well, I believe that practitioners and patients alike are often guilty of the same forces. If we're working as a medical doctor, our confirmation bias means that we'll focus on the evidence that supports our view, and the patients we've successfully treated, to reinforce it. The same thing happens for alternative practitioners. We might treat three people with a condition, and then find ourselves talking to colleagues and future patients about only the one patient who did improve.

This confirmation bias effect is further compounded by the fact that those we help tend to keep coming to see us, and those we don't, do not. So we find ourselves spending a disproportionate amount of time around the very people who confirm the bias of our perspective.

The same effect happens for those on the healing journey. Patients look for the evidence that supports the path they currently believe in, and some will also become like religious zealots, defending a particular methodology against others. The danger is that we increasingly become less focused on the facts and instead are pulled by the ideas that make us feel safer and more comfortable in our current choices.

Protecting Against Confirmation Bias

The consequences of this confirmation bias effect can be far-reaching, and as either practitioners or sufferers, we need to be diligent in protecting against it. At the OHC, we have specific internal processes designed to mitigate its effect. For example, each practitioner has internal case reviews of their client base to make sure people aren't slipping through the net. And we have an ongoing review process to make sure that we stay up to date with those patients who aren't in regular consultations.

As a fatigue sufferer, I'd advise you not to be afraid to ask challenging questions of your practitioners, and be on the lookout for anyone who has tunnel vision and only looks at cases from a single perspective. And don't be afraid to challenge your *own* beliefs and assumptions at any stage, either. If something's built on solid evidence, after the application of some cautious scrutiny, it'll still be true.

Do Your Research

I've always been a great believer in providing as much free information as possible online, and I must have released more than 1,000 videos on YouTube over the years. I love the fact that I can spend 10 minutes making a video which can then potentially be seen by thousands of people. And I'm not alone – these days, practitioners are increasingly sharing their ideas online for free.

Try everything you can to take advantage of the free information provided by practitioners – use it to check both their philosophical approach and how they resonate with you as people. Don't be afraid to make the most of any free exploration process they offer; for example, at the OHC we have a team of highly experienced New Patient Coordinators who will happily spend considerable time on the phone with prospective patients, answering questions for free. Always take the time to do your research before committing resources toward any particular path, and remember to trust your instincts – they're usually correct.

Preparing for a Consultation

Having just an hour or so with a practitioner can feel like a tiny amount of time when so much is going on in our body and mind. This is why careful preparation for consultations is critical. As simple as the following suggestions might sound, you'd be amazed how often people fail to follow them:

1. Write down your questions in advance. There is no guarantee there'll be time to ask all of your questions (particularly if they are driven by an anxiety pattern, i.e. they're endless), and indeed, doing so could be a poor use of consultation time because it distracts from the key focuses, which a skilled practitioner will be able to navigate. But equally, spending half the session feeling frustrated because you had an important question that you can't remember isn't a good use of time and focus either.

2. Email your questions, and an update of any changes since the last consultation, to your practitioner in advance. Although some practitioners might not be willing to read emails ahead of a session, even if they read your questions at the start of the session, it can be an immensely helpful way of maximizing time by giving them a quick overview of where you're at and what's happening.

3. If you're having a session in person, be sure to arrive early so you have time to settle into the space and don't spend half the time flustered and trying to find your words. To get the most out of consultations, you need to support yourself in being in the best state possible, given your current circumstances.

4. If you're having a session online, don't schedule it directly against other meetings on either side, and make sure you're in a quiet place where you feel you can talk freely and safely.

How To Get the Most Out of Sessions

When actually in sessions with a practitioner, be careful not to overly control the agenda. A natural byproduct of an anxiety pattern, or indeed being in the maladaptive stress response, is that we try to think our way to a feeling of safety. This means that we have endless questions, many of which are driven by an underlying feeling of stress and anxiety. The reality is though, no sooner have these questions been answered than another dozen may surface.

An experienced practitioner will have their own agenda for structuring sessions and usually they'll do their best work when we let them follow this. That's not to say you should ignore your own instincts if you feel they're going in the wrong direction, and it's a delicate balance between being passive and trying to take control.

The ideal is to be an active participant who lets the practitioner do their job. This can sometimes mean being open to hearing things we don't want to hear, and equally, speaking our own truths when the practitioner might not want to hear them. There is no perfect science to it, but being sensitive to these very challenges is a great start.

When practitioner and patient are working together in harmony, both playing their roles as skillfully as they can, it's a beautiful and potent partnership. When they're not, it can be the most frustrating thing in the world.

Ultimately, when it comes down to it, you have to learn to listen to and trust your intuition. How you feel with someone is important information, and to truly commit to a process, it has to feel right to you. Our intuition doesn't always give us convenient answers, and having the courage to act on what we believe to be truth to us can be an important turning point in the healing journey. This is particularly true for those who have strong helper patterns and tend to make the needs of others more important than their own, and that can include a practitioner whose time they are paying for.

What to Do When Things Go Wrong

If you feel strongly that things aren't going right in a particular therapeutic relationship, I cannot emphasize enough the importance of raising your concerns. Any professional practitioner will be open to hearing what you have to say, and if they aren't, that alone probably tells you all you need to know about your compatibility with them.

In my experience some of the most important therapeutic breakthroughs have happened when a patient has had the courage to bring a concern to the table and together we've explored it, only to find a piece of information that was missing, or a new path for how things needed to move forward.

That's not to say that the therapeutic relationship is always meant to be a smooth or a simple one. Sometimes, particularly when we're working on the psychology side, we can hit challenging territory where people are being forced to see things about themselves and their lives that are confronting and uncomfortable. But even then this should be done with care, compassion, and kindness.

All this said, getting the most out of consultations is an art, and we get better at it with practice. Be gentle with yourself and remember that a practitioner's job is to help you; if they're not doing that, you're within your rights to ask probing questions.

Now that we've explored the key elements of decoding your fatigue and have mapped your path to recovery, we're going to bring it all together. It's time for us to create a plan for your recovery.

Chapter 18

CREATE YOUR RECOVERY PLAN

Wow, you've done it! I know that this has been an intense journey at times, so congratulations for getting this far. At this point, you won't be alone if you're feeling a combination of excitement at the possibility of things changing and a sense of confusion and overwhelm about where to start.

So, I have a question for you – how do you eat an elephant?

Well, assuming you're not a vegetarian or vegan, and that you're into exotic types of meat, the answer is simply 'one mouthful at a time.'

Just as you can't eat an elephant in one sitting, you can't put into action every aspect of this book in one go, and neither should you try. Our job together in this chapter is to come up with a plan for where to start and how.

12 Steps to Decode Your Fatigue and Support Healing

To do this, we're going to review the 12 steps, or lessons, we've covered in the book:

1. Take responsibility

2. Get an accurate diagnosis

3. Understand the role of your mitochondria

4. Understand your personality

5. Create an environment for healing

6. Get in a healing state

7. Optimize your digestion

8. Balance your hormones

9. Support your immune system

10. Discover your baseline and learn to pace

11. Optimize your food

12. Manage your team

Step 1: Take responsibility

Whether it seems fair or not, you *have* to take responsibility for your healing journey. Just like the turning point I had in the conversation with my uncle, I hope that a similar realization has happened for you. If your life is to change, you're the one who's going to have to change it.

Step 2: Get an accurate diagnosis

There is a reason I labored this point in Chapter 2: there are a number of medically understood issues that could be causing your fatigue and the only way to be sure they aren't playing a role is to see a suitably qualified medical doctor. Some of these could also be warning signs of potentially life-threatening conditions and they'll require swift medical attention. So, as I said earlier, *do not take this warning lightly.*

However, if your diagnosis *is* one of fatigue, chronic fatigue, ME, post-viral fatigue, fibromyalgia, and so on, then I don't really believe you have a diagnosis. You have a name for a collection of symptoms but, as we discussed, it tells you nothing about the reason those symptoms are there in the first place.

Step 3: Understand the role of your mitochondria

Your next step is to understand the role of your mitochondria. Remember, your fatigue has a biochemical explanation and is down to your cellular energy production. Understanding the key principles of this process is critical for decoding your fatigue, and it can be a huge relief to realize there is a real biological basis to your fatigue.

Step 4: Understand your personality

In the first chapter of Part II, we explored the five energy depleting personality patterns – the achiever, helper, anxiety, perfectionist, and controller. You may have identified one or two of them as your own pattern, and you might also have recognized all of them. The key here is that you practice catching these patterns when they're playing out, as we discussed in Chapter 15, because left unchecked, these patterns will not only trigger your maladaptive stress response, they'll also constantly undermine your attempts to better manage your activity levels.

Step 5: Create an environment for healing

Your next step is to work on creating a better environment for healing. The loads of your past may well have played a key role in causing your fatigue, and you may need to deal with the ongoing impacts and effects of that. Equally, if you have too many loads on your boat right now, then your body won't have the right environment to support your healing.

Step 6: Get in a healing state

This brings us to our next step: for your body to heal, it has to be in a healing state. As we discussed in Chapter 8, and revisited in Chapter 15, it's crucial that you work to calm your nervous system. Sometimes the impact of this can be very dramatic, and at the very least, a robust recovery won't be possible without this step.

Step 7: Optimize your digestion

We then turned our attention to your digestive function in Chapter 9. If your body isn't breaking down and absorbing energy from your food, then your mitochondria don't stand a chance of working properly. We explored a number of possible issues that could be playing a role in your digestive system. Working with a skilled practitioner here may be an important key.

Step 8: Balance your hormones

Next, we looked at your hormones in Chapter 10, primarily focusing on your adrenal glands. When you're under stress of any sort, your adrenals work harder. When your mitochondria aren't producing enough energy, it's the job of your adrenals to fill the gap. Over time, the effect of all this is that your adrenals become dysregulated. It can be tempting to use stimulants to keep you going, but that will just make everything worse.

Step 9: Support your immune system

In Chapter 11, we explored your immune function, and I made the point that fatigue is rarely caused by a single viral overload. Equally, if your immune system is overworking, it'll significantly impact your energy levels. We explored some key principles around possible viral causes, toxic mold, and Lyme disease and coinfections. If any of these ring true for you, then again, working with a suitably skilled practitioner will be crucial.

Step 10: Discover your baseline and learn to pace

As we turned our attention to fatigue map 2, your path to recovery, in chapters 13 and 14 we explored the critical importance of listening to your body, discovering your baseline, and learning to pace. We also explored the three stages of recovery. It can be tempting to ignore the challenging steps I've asked you to take in these chapters, and hope that by fixing other elements you can keep going as you are. I'm afraid this logic is flawed. You simply cannot push your body to recovery – you have to give it the rest it needs. Everything we're doing here isn't about 'fixing' your body: it's about creating the environment and giving it the support it needs to heal itself.

Step 11: Optimize your food

In Chapter 16, we explored the key dietary changes you can make to help support your healing. This built on what we explored in Chapter 9; and remember: it's about making consistent, sustainable changes, not getting things perfect.

Step 12: Manage your team

Finally, in Chapter 17 we explored how to find the right practitioners, and how best to manage your relationship with them in a proactive way. Recovery is rarely something we do on our own, and the better we can manage those relationships, the more effective they'll be.

Setting Your Recovery Goals

Where do you begin with the 12-step plan? Well, my recommendation would be to start by working through the free companion course that accompanies this book – access it at www.alexhoward.com/fatigue. You'll hear directly from many of the people whose case studies we've explored, which will bring their inspiring recovery stories to life. You can also get started with the guided meditation and the simple recipe plans.

I also strongly encourage you to go back and reread chapters 13 and 14. Getting your activity levels right and establishing the stage of recovery you're at are utterly crucial to plotting your next steps forward. Remember, what works for someone at one stage can make things worse at another.

To help put together some of these changes, it can be helpful to have a few goals to focus on. As we explored in Chapter 12, the mindset chapter, you have to be committed and motivated on the healing path. But how do you do that in a way that doesn't trigger more achiever pattern and trying to do too much, too quickly?

The secret is not to set goals for how much activity you'll do, or when certain symptoms will have improved. These are things that you might be able to influence indirectly, but they aren't things whose outcome you can control, and attempting to do so will likely cause you to do too much.

What's far more helpful is to set goals around the habits and behaviors you need to change, which will in turn help create the environment internally and externally that best supports things moving forward. So, rather than setting a goal of how much activity you're going to do in the coming month, set a goal of committing to a daily mediation practice of a certain duration, or the foods you're going to change or introduce into your diet.

Now, given that the achiever pattern is rather widespread in the fatigue population, try to be extremely cautious here that you commit to things in a way that'll actually be helpful. If I had to do my recovery journey again, one of the things I'd most definitely change would be the intensity with which I approached my healing. Yes, a commitment to getting well was critical, and without that conversation with my uncle I honestly believe I might not be here today. But equally, for the body to heal, it has to be in a healing state, and this isn't happening when we're constantly pushing too hard.

What Are Your Recovery Goals?

Here are a few examples of the recovery goals you might set. Come up with your own ideas and pick 1–3 of them that you're going to get started with right away.

1. I'm going to commit 30 minutes a day for the next week to working through the Decode Your Fatigue companion course.

2. I'm going to listen to the guided meditation in the companion course once a day for the next month.

3. By the end of this week I'll have reached out to a practitioner to take the next step on healing my digestion.

What's Life Trying to Teach You?

Sometimes your recovery goals might be simple behavioral changes, such as those we've just talked about, but other times they may be more fundamental. Perhaps a key part of your problem is that your life has been set up in a way that's not only a major factor in your getting ill but, based on what we've explored together, is also clearly a major obstacle to your healing.

I'm afraid this is where we get into some hard and unforgiving truths. Your healing might involve some very difficult life changes. Perhaps you've been in a long-term relationship that's toxic and your fatigue is your body's way of telling you to get away. Or perhaps you're pursuing a career that you hate; maybe it was always your parents' dream and not yours, and your fatigue is your body's way of trying to communicate with you.

And this is where we get to perhaps the most controversial statement I've made in this book: perhaps your being ill is happening for a reason. It might be that your body isn't just a broken engine but actually has a deep wisdom worth listening to. When we're at our lowest point, it might be impossible to hear this wisdom, but I've seen it happen countless times. On the other side of their fatigue journey, many people end up with happier and better lives than they would otherwise have had. To illustrate this point, I'm going to end this chapter by telling you the story of my sister-in-law.

It was Christmas 2012 and my wife Tania was very recently pregnant with our second daughter. We were looking forward to a quiet and relaxed family Christmas, and as I enjoyed the slowing down of a hectic work schedule, I was becoming aware that Tania's younger sister, Violet, was struggling with her health.

Tania had always been very close to her sister. When Violet had found out we were having our first daughter, Marli, she'd moved her entire life back to the UK, after living for almost a decade in Australia, to be close to us. Because Violet had moved back only recently at that time, I was just beginning to get to know her.

In the previous few months, Violet had badly broken her foot after missing a step while walking down some stairs and had suffered a severe lung infection that was refusing to clear. Over the Christmas period, we became so concerned about Violet that I took her to the hospital's emergency department on one occasion, and Tania and I cancelled our New Year's holiday so we could stay home and look after her.

At the time, I didn't think much of it – it just seemed like an acute episode of temporary health difficulties that needed some time to heal. A few months later, although Violet's foot was healing and her lungs were slowly on the mend, something was still not right. Of particular concern was the fact she was suffering from an almost overwhelming fatigue, to the point where she'd had to give up a job she loved – working as a social worker supporting families in central London who were experiencing extreme poverty.

Having attended several further medical appointments with Violet, including one where I almost ended up in an argument with a top consultant who'd had the nerve to tell her she was most likely just depressed, it became clear that she was suffering from post-viral fatigue syndrome. At the time, Tania and I were in the process of moving into a larger house to accommodate our expanding family, and we invited Violet to live with us for a few months while she regained her strength.

As the months passed, my assumption was that Violet would soon feel a lot better and move on with her life. But she didn't. In fact, things got worse. Within a few months of moving in with us, she was almost entirely housebound, and at times we even had to cook meals for her.

At this point, we all started to take things rather more seriously. Violet started working with the practitioner teams at the OHC, and although there were some small initial gains, along with a stabilization of the serious crashes she'd been experiencing, she didn't make the progress I generally saw with patients.

At the OHC we've always said that our approach evolves the most through the patients with whom we struggle; however, I'd never anticipated that one of the patients I'd learn the most from would be my sister-in-law, in my own house. We used to joke that Violet was receiving the money-can't-buy 'deluxe' OHC package, which includes moving in with the founder. However, clinical learnings aside, it was increasingly concerning for me to see the approach I'd spent my adult life developing failing to help someone I loved.

Around two years into Violet's illness, one of our nutrition team raised some questions about some of her immune markers in a recent round of blood tests. There was nothing conclusive but her system did appear to be fighting something. It was then suggested that Violet might have Lyme disease.

I'd been aware of Lyme disease for a number of years. Indeed, I recalled Niki saying to me several years previously, in her usual passionate way, 'Alex, I'm telling you, this is going to be the next major challenge for the fatigue community.' But if I'm honest, I knew less about it than I should have, and the OHC's protocols for working with it were at a very elementary stage.

In the months that followed, Violet and I went on a major learning curve together. Violet threw an enormous amount of her limited energy into researching Lyme and the different treatment paths. We both quickly realized it was a very young area of science and a perfect example of both the conflict between the approaches of conventional and functional medicine and their potential to work in harmony together. Indeed, it's partly down to Violet's healing journey that the OHC's approach to working with Lyme has developed in the years since.

During Violet's time living with us, she took up sketching, initially just to help pass the day. Sometimes she spent just a few minutes a day on it, but in time her projects became a little more elaborate. Because her bedroom was at the top of the house, many months went by when I didn't see what she was up to with her art. That was until my birthday came around. Violet was immensely grateful for the depth of support that Tania and I had given her and she'd wanted to find a way to thank me. And so her first major drawing with charcoal was a gift for my birthday.

When Violet gave me the piece, I was literally speechless. It was a staggeringly intricate and deeply moving portrait of a beautifully wrinkled old lady. It has pride of place in our living room to this day. On the back of that, I commissioned Violet to do her next piece as a gift for a close friend of mine, and before she knew it, things snowballed.

In the years that followed, as Violet continued to recover, her life took an entirely new direction. Indeed, art went from being a trusted friend on her healing journey to becoming her means of supporting herself. As Violet continued to push boundaries with both her healing and her artwork, her new career started to gather its own momentum. By talking openly about her healing journey, Violet also brought an authenticity and depth to her work.

These days, Violet has an amazing career as an artist and has recently exhibited in London and Oman. She truly loves her work, which integrates her passion for conservation with art, and she lives a wonderful life.

Looking back, Violet's convinced that if it hadn't been for those immensely challenging years suffering from Lyme disease, she would never have discovered and cultivated her love of art. It had been a very painful journey but also a worthwhile one that she wouldn't change. (In the companion course, you can watch an interview we recorded of Violet's story, and also see the artwork she gifted me for my birthday.)

It might be a very hard thing to hear, but perhaps this is all happening to you for a reason. That reason might not become clear right away;

however, I know from experience that if nothing else, looking for the positives is a more empowering choice to make.

Ultimately, your healing journey isn't only a physical and emotional one – it's also a journey for your soul. Trust the process, listen to your body, and you might be amazed at where it takes you.

▪▪ REFERENCES ▪▪

Chapter 1: Radical Responsibility

1. Arroll, M.A. and Howard, A. (2013), 'The letting go, the building up [and] the gradual process of rebuilding: Identity change and post-traumatic growth in myalgic encephalomyelitis/chronic fatigue syndrome': www. tandfonline.com/doi/full/10.1080/08870446.2012.721882

2. Arroll, M.A. and Howard, A. (2012), 'A preliminary prospective study of nutritional, psychological and combined therapies for myalgic encephalomyelitis/chronic fatigue syndrome (ME/CFS) in a private care setting': www.ncbi.nlm.nih.gov/pubmed/23166120

3. Arroll, M.A., et al. (2014), 'Pilot study investigating the utility of a specialized online symptom management program for individuals with myalgic encephalomyelitis/chronic fatigue syndrome as compared to an online meditation program': www.dovepress.com/pilot-study-investigating-the-utility-of-a-specialized-online-symptom--peer-reviewed-article-PRBM

Chapter 2: Why Conventional Medicine Is Baffled by Fatigue

4. Wortman, M.S.H., et al. (2018), 'Cost-effectiveness of interventions for medically unexplained symptoms: A systematic review': www.ncbi.nlm. nih.gov/pmc/articles/PMC6188754/

5. Burton, C. (2003), 'Beyond somatisation: a review of the understanding and treatment of medically unexplained physical symptoms (MUPS)': www.ncbi.nlm.nih.gov/pmc/articles/PMC1314551/

6.   The Medical Staff of the Royal Free Hospital (1957), 'An outbreak of encephalomyelitis in the Royal Free Hospital Group, London, in 1955': www.ncbi.nlm.nih.gov/pubmed/13472002

7.   Ramsay, A.M. (1965), 'Hysteria and "Royal Free Disease"': www.ncbi. nlm.nih.gov/pmc/articles/PMC1847119/?page=1

8.   Ramsay, A.M., et al. (1977), 'Icelandic disease (benign myalgic encephalomyelitis or Royal Free disease)': www.ncbi.nlm.nih.gov/ pubmed/861618

9.   Ramsay, A.M. (1978), 'Epidemic neuromyasthenia 1955–1978': www. ncbi.nlm.nih.gov/pubmed/746017

10. Pasteur (1881), 'On the Germ Theory': www.ncbi.nlm.nih.gov/ pubmed/17830637

11. Smith, K.A. (2012), 'Louis Pasteur, the father of immunology?': www. ncbi.nlm.nih.gov/pubmed/22566949

12. Cortes Rivera, M., et al. (2019), 'Myalgic Encephalomyelitis/Chronic Fatigue Syndrome: A Comprehensive Review': www.ncbi.nlm.nih.gov/ pubmed/31394725

13. Sweetman, E., et al. (2019), 'Current Research Provides Insight into the Biological Basis and Diagnostic Potential for Myalgic Encephalomyelitis/ Chronic Fatigue Syndrome (ME/CFS)': www.ncbi.nlm.nih.gov/ pubmed/31295930

14. Underhill, R.A. (2015), 'Myalgic encephalomyelitis, chronic fatigue syndrome: An infectious disease': http://dx.doi.org/10.1016/j. mehy.2015.10.011

15. Rowe, P.C., et al. (2017), 'Myalgic Encephalomyelitis/Chronic Fatigue Syndrome Diagnosis and Management in Young People: A Primer': www.ncbi.nlm.nih.gov/pubmed/28674681

16. McEvedy, C.P. and Beard, A.W. (1970), 'Concept of benign myalgic encephalomyelitis': www.ncbi.nlm.nih.gov/pubmed/5411596

17. McManimen, S., et al. (2019), 'Dismissing chronic illness: A qualitative analysis of negative health care experiences': www.ncbi.nlm.nih.gov/ pubmed/30829147

18. Friedman, K.J. (2019), 'Advances in ME/CFS: Past, Present, and Future': www.ncbi.nlm.nih.gov/pubmed/31058116

19. Centers for Disease Control and Prevention (2020), 'Myalgic Encephalomyelitis/Chronic Fatigue Syndrome (ME/CFS)': www.cdc.gov/me-cfs/index.html

20. Raine, R., et al. (2004), 'General practitioners' perceptions of chronic fatigue syndrome and beliefs about its management, compared with irritable bowel syndrome: qualitative study': www.ncbi.nlm.nih.gov/pmc/articles/PMC420289/

21. Lian, O.S. and Robson, C. (2017), '"It's incredible how much I've had to fight"'; negotiating medical uncertainty in clinical encounters': www.ncbi.nlm.nih.gov/pubmed/29063801

22. Collin, S.M. and Crawley, E. (2017), 'Specialist treatment of chronic fatigue syndrome/ME: a cohort study among adult patients in England': www.ncbi.nlm.nih.gov/pubmed/28709432

23. Maizes, V., et al. (2009), 'Integrative Medicine and Patient-Centered Care': www.sciencedirect.com/science/article/abs/pii/S1550830709002341?via%3Dihub

24. Ali, A. and Katz, D.L. (2015), 'Disease Prevention and Health Promotion: How Integrative Medicine Fits': www.ncbi.nlm.nih.gov/pubmed/26477898

25. Bland, J. (2015), 'Functional Medicine: An Operating System for Integrative Medicine': http://www.ncbi.nlm.nih.gov/pubmed/26770161

26. National Institute of Clinical Excellence (NICE) (2007), 'Chronic fatigue syndrome/myalgic encephalomyelitis (or encephalopathy): diagnosis and management of chronic fatigue syndrome/myalgic encephalomyelitis (or encephalopathy) in adults and children': http://guidance.nice.org.uk/CG53/Guidance/pdf/English

27. Baker, R. and Shaw, E.J. (2007), 'Guidelines: Diagnosis and management of chronic fatigue syndrome or myalgic encephalomyelitis (or encephalopathy): Summary of NICE guidance', *British Medical Journal*, 335(7617): 446–8.

28. Jones, J.F. et al. (2009), 'An evaluation of exclusionary medical/psychiatric conditions in the definition of chronic fatigue syndrome': https://pubmed.ncbi.nlm.nih.gov/19818157/

29. Fukuda, K. et al. (1994), 'The chronic fatigue syndrome: a comprehensive approach to its definition and study': www.ncbi.nlm.nih. gov/pubmed/7978722

30. Brurberg, K.G. et al. (2014), 'Case definitions for chronic fatigue syndrome/myalgic encephalomyelitis (CFS/ME): a systematic review': www.ncbi.nlm.nih.gov/pubmed/24508851

31. Brimmer, D.J. et al. (2013), 'A pilot registry of unexplained fatiguing illnesses and chronic fatigue syndrome': www.ncbi.nlm.nih.gov/ pubmed/23915640

32. Bansal, A.S. (2016), 'Investigating unexplained fatigue in general practice with a particular focus on CFS/ME': www.ncbi.nlm.nih.gov/ pubmed/27436349

33. Strand, E.B. et al. (2019), 'Myalgic encephalomyelitis/chronic fatigue Syndrome (ME/CFS): Investigating care practices pointed out to disparities in diagnosis and treatment across European Union': www. ncbi.nlm.nih.gov/pubmed/31805176

34. Cohen, H. (2017), 'Controversies and challenges in fibromyalgia: a review and a proposal': www.ncbi.nlm.nih.gov/pubmed/28458723

35. Arnold, L.M. et al. (2016), 'Fibromyalgia and Chronic Pain Syndromes: A White Paper Detailing Current Challenges in the Field': www.ncbi. nlm.nih.gov/pubmed/27022674

36. Garcia-Monco, J.C. and Benach, J.L. (2019), 'Lyme Neuroborreliosis: Clinical Outcomes, Controversy, Pathogenesis, and Polymicrobial Infections': www.ncbi.nlm.nih.gov/pubmed/30536421

37. Jaulhac, B., et al. (2019), 'Lyme borreliosis and other tick-borne diseases. Guidelines from the French scientific societies (II). Biological diagnosis, treatment, persistent symptoms after documented or suspected Lyme borreliosis': www.sciencedirect.com/science/article/ pii/S0399077X19301313?via%3Dihub

38. Rauer, S., et al. (2018), 'Lyme Neuroborreliosis': www.ncbi.nlm.nih. gov/pubmed/30573008

39. Baker, P.J. (2020), 'A Review of Antibiotic-Tolerant Persisters and Their Relevance to Post-treatment Lyme Disease Symptoms': www.ncbi.nlm. nih.gov/pubmed/31926865

Chapter 3: How Your Body Creates Energy

40. Morris, G. and Maes, M. (2014), 'Mitochondrial dysfunctions in Myalgic Encephalomyelitis/chronic fatigue syndrome explained by activated immuno-inflammatory, oxidative and nitrosative stress pathways', *Metabolic Brain Disease*, 29(1):19–36.

41. Zarębska, A.E., et al. (2018), 'Plasma Nucleotide Dynamics during Exercise and Recovery in Highly Trained Athletes and Recreationally Active Individuals': www.hindawi.com/journals/bmri/2018/4081802

42. Nacul, L., et al. (2019), 'Evidence of Clinical Pathology Abnormalities in People with Myalgic Encephalomyelitis/Chronic Fatigue Syndrome (ME/CFS) from an Analytic Cross-Sectional Study': www.ncbi.nlm.nih.gov/pubmed/30974900

43. Twisk, F.N.M. (2015), 'Accurate diagnosis of myalgic encephalomyelitis and chronic fatigue syndrome based upon objective test methods for characteristic symptoms': www.pubmedcentral.nih.gov/articlerender.fcgi?artid=4482824&tool=pmcentrez&rendertype=abstract

44. VanNess, J.M., et al. (2010), 'Postexertional Malaise in Women with Chronic Fatigue Syndrome': www.liebertpub.com/doi/10.1089/jwh.2009.1507

45. Holtzman, C., et al. (2019), 'Assessment of Post-Exertional Malaise (PEM) in Patients with Myalgic Encephalomyelitis (ME) and Chronic Fatigue Syndrome (CFS): A Patient-Driven Survey': www.mdpi.com/2075-4418/9/1/26

46. Bou-Holaigah, I. (1995), 'The Relationship Between Neurally Mediated Hypotension and the Chronic Fatigue Syndrome': http://jama.jamanetwork.com/article.aspx?articleid=389684

47. Ocon, A.J., et al. (2012), 'Increasing orthostatic stress impairs neurocognitive functioning in chronic fatigue syndrome with postural tachycardia syndrome': www.ncbi.nlm.nih.gov/pubmed/21919887

48. Chu, L., et al. (2018), 'Deconstructing post-exertional malaise in myalgic encephalomyelitis/chronic fatigue syndrome: A patient-centered, cross-sectional survey': www.ncbi.nlm.nih.gov/pubmed/29856774

49. Arroll, M.A., et al. (2014), 'The delayed fatigue effect in myalgic encephalomyelitis/chronic fatigue syndrome (ME/CFS)': www.tandfonline.com/doi/abs/10.1080/21641846.2014.892755

50. Cvejic, E., et al. (2017), 'Autonomic nervous system function, activity patterns, and sleep after physical or cognitive challenge in people with chronic fatigue syndrome': www.ncbi.nlm.nih.gov/pubmed/29167053

51. Nijs, J., et al. (2012), 'In the mind or in the brain? Scientific evidence for central sensitisation in chronic fatigue syndrome': www.ncbi.nlm.nih.gov/pubmed/21793823

52. Myhill, S., et al. (2009), 'Chronic fatigue syndrome and mitochondrial dysfunction': www.ncbi.nlm.nih.gov/pmc/articles/PMC2680051/

53. Booth, N.E., et al. (2012), 'Mitochondrial dysfunction and the pathophysiology of Myalgic Encephalomyelitis/Chronic Fatigue Syndrome (ME/CFS)': www.ncbi.nlm.nih.gov/pubmed/22837795

54. Nicolson, G.L. (2014), 'Mitochondrial dysfunction and chronic disease: Treatment with natural supplements', *Integrative Medicine*, 13(4): 35–43.

55. Werbach, M. (2000), 'Nutritional strategies for treating chronic fatigue syndrome': https://pubmed.ncbi.nlm.nih.gov/10767667/

Chapter 4: How Your Mind and Emotions Affect Fatigue

56. Barnden, L.R., et al. (2015), 'Evidence in chronic fatigue syndrome for severity-dependent upregulation of prefrontal myelination that is independent of anxiety and depression': http://doi.wiley.com/10.1002/nbm.3261

57. Christley, Y., et al. (2013), 'The Neuropsychiatric and Neuropsychological Features of Chronic Fatigue Syndrome: Revisiting the Enigma': https://pubmed.ncbi.nlm.nih.gov/23440559/?dopt=Abstract

58. Griffith, J.P. and Zarrouf, F.A. (2008), 'A systematic review of chronic fatigue syndrome: don't assume it's depression': www.pubmedcentral.nih.gov/articlerender.fcgi?artid=2292451&tool=pmcentrez&rendertype=abstract

59. Zschucke, E., et al. (2013), 'Exercise and physical activity in mental disorders: clinical and experimental evidence': www.ncbi.nlm.nih.gov/pubmed/23412549J

60. Wegner, M., et al. (2020), 'Systematic Review of Meta-Analyses: Exercise Effects on Depression in Children and Adolescents': www.ncbi.nlm.nih.gov/pubmed/32210847

61. Schuch, B.F. et al. (2016), 'Exercise as a Treatment for Depression: A Meta-Analysis Adjusting for Publication Bias': https://pubmed.ncbi. nlm.nih.gov/26978184/

62. Kimberlee, R., et al. (2013), 'Measuring the economic impact of the wellspring healthy living centre's social prescribing wellbeing programme for low level mental health issues encountered by GP services': https:// uwe-repository.worktribe.com/output/926277

63. Bjørkum, T., et al. (2009), 'Patients' experience with treatment of chronic fatigue syndrome': www.ncbi.nlm.nih.gov/pubmed/19521443

64. Geraghty, K., et al. (2019), 'Myalgic encephalomyelitis/chronic fatigue syndrome patients reports of symptom changes following cognitive behavioural therapy, graded exercise therapy and pacing treatments: Analysis of a primary survey compared with secondary surveys': https:// pubmed.ncbi.nlm.nih.gov/28847166/

65. Vink, M. and Vink-Niese, A. (2018), 'Graded exercise therapy for myalgic encephalomyelitis/chronic fatigue syndrome is not effective and unsafe. Re-analysis of a Cochrane review': www.ncbi.nlm.nih.gov/ pubmed/30305916

66. Kindlon, T. (2017), 'Do Graded Activity Therapies Cause Harm in Chronic Fatigue Syndrome?' https://pubmed.ncbi.nlm.nih. gov/28805516/

67. Taylor, A.K., et al. (2017), '"It's personal to me": A qualitative study of depression in young people with CFS/ME': https://pubmed.ncbi.nlm. nih.gov/27742756/

68. Kiecolt-Glaser, J.K., et al. (1986), 'Modulation of Cellular Immunity in Medical Students': http://pni.osumc.edu/KG Publications %28pdf%29/013.pdf

69. Gouin, J-P. and Kiecolt-Glaser, J.K. (2011), 'The impact of psychological stress on wound healing: methods and mechanisms': www.ncbi.nlm.nih. gov/pubmed/21094925

70. Kiecolt-Glaser, J.K., et al. (1995), 'Slowing of wound healing by psychological stress': https://pubmed.ncbi.nlm.nih.gov/7475659/

71. Naviaux, R.K. (2014), 'Metabolic features of the cell danger response': www.sciencedirect.com/science/article/pii/S1567724913002390

72. Naviaux, R.K. (2019), 'Perspective: Cell Danger Response Biology—The New Science that Connects Environmental Health with Mitochondria and the Rising Tide of Chronic Illness': www.sciencedirect.com/science/article/pii/S1567724919302922?via%3Dihub

73. Naviaux, R.K., et al. (2016), 'Metabolic features of chronic fatigue syndrome': https://pubmed.ncbi.nlm.nih.gov/27573827/

Chapter 5: A New Model for Understanding Fatigue

74. Belcourt, S., et al. (2001), 'A twin Study of Chronic Fatigue': www.academia.edu/2725172/

75. Perez, M., et al. (2019), 'Genetic Predisposition for Immune System, Hormone, and Metabolic Dysfunction in Myalgic Encephalomyelitis/Chronic Fatigue Syndrome: A Pilot Study': www.ncbi.nlm.nih.gov/pmc/articles/PMC6542994/

76. Fitzgerald, K. (not yet published), 'Methylation Diet and Lifestyle Study': https://clinicaltrials.gov/ct2/show/study/NCT03472820

Chapter 6: The Personality of Fatigue

77. Tack, M. (2019), 'Letter to the Editor (March 3, 2019) concerning the paper "The relationship between chronic fatigue syndrome, burnout, job satisfaction, social support and age among academics at a tertiary institution"': www.journalssystem.com/ijomeh/Letter-to-the-editor-concerning-the-paper-The-relationship-between-chronic-fatigue,105960,0,2.html

78. Alderman, C. (1990), 'Yuppie 'flu – a real illness': http://journals.rcni.com/doi/10.7748/ns.4.49.18.s33

Chapter 7: Understanding the Loads on Your Body

79. Felitti, V.J., et al. (2019), 'Reprint of: Relationship of Childhood Abuse and Household Dysfunction to Many of the Leading Causes of Death in Adults: The Adverse Childhood Experiences (ACE) Study': https://linkinghub.elsevier.com/retrieve/pii/S0749379719301436

80. Finkelhor, D., et al. (2015), 'A revised inventory of Adverse Childhood Experiences': www.sciencedirect.com/science/article/abs/pii/S0145213415002409?via%3Dihub

81. Afifi, T.O., et al. (2020), 'Confirmatory factor analysis of adverse childhood experiences (ACEs) among a community-based sample of parents and adolescents': www.ncbi.nlm.nih.gov/pubmed/32316954BMC

82. Shalev, I., et al. (2020), 'Investigating the impact of early-life adversity on physiological, immune, and gene expression responses to acute stress: A pilot feasibility study': www.ncbi.nlm.nih.gov/pmc/articles/PMC7122782/

83. Gerritsen, L., et al. (2017), 'HPA Axis Genes, and Their Interaction with Childhood Maltreatment, are Related to Cortisol Levels and Stress-Related Phenotypes': www.ncbi.nlm.nih.gov/pubmed/28589964 2017

84. Steenkamp, M.M., et al. (2017), 'Predictors of PTSD 40 years after combat: Findings from the National Vietnam Veterans longitudinal study': http://doi.wiley.com/10.1002/da.22628

85. Howley, E. (2019), 'Statistics on PTSD in Veterans': https://health.usnews.com/conditions/mental-health/ptsd/articles/ptsd-veterans-statistics

Chapter 8: Are You In a Healing State?

86. Chu, B., et al. (2020), 'Physiology, Stress Reaction': www.ncbi.nlm.nih.gov/pubmed/31082164

87. Porges, S.W. (2001), 'The polyvagal theory: phylogenetic substrates of a social nervous system': www.sciencedirect.com/science/article/abs/pii/S0167876001001623?via%3Dihub

88. Porges, S.W. (2009), 'The polyvagal theory: new insights into adaptive reactions of the autonomic nervous system': www.ncbi.nlm.nih.gov/pubmed/19376991

89. Zimmermann, A., et al. (2014), 'When less is more: hormesis against stress and disease': http://microbialcell.com/researcharticles/when-less-is-more-hormesis-against-stress-and-disease/

90. van Oort, J., et al. (2020), 'Absence of default mode downregulation in response to a mild psychological stressor marks stress-vulnerability

across diverse psychiatric disorders': www.sciencedirect.com/science/article/pii/S2213158220300152

91. Kinlein, S.A., et al. (2015), 'Dysregulated hypothalamic-pituitary-adrenal axis function contributes to altered endocrine and neurobehavioral responses to acute stress': www.ncbi.nlm.nih.gov/pubmed/25821436

92. Dunlavey, C.J. (2018), 'Introduction to the Hypothalamic-Pituitary-Adrenal Axis: Healthy and Dysregulated Stress Responses, Developmental Stress and Neurodegeneration': www.ncbi.nlm.nih.gov/pubmed/30057514

Chapter 9: Your Digestive System – Breaking Down Your Energy Source

93. Sender, R., et al. (2016), 'Revised Estimates for the Number of Human and Bacteria Cells in the Body': www.ncbi.nlm.nih.gov/pmc/articles/PMC4991899/

94. Belkaid, Y. and Hand, T.W. (2014), 'Role of the microbiota in immunity and inflammation': www.ncbi.nlm.nih.gov/pubmed/24679531

95. Carabotti, M., et al. (2015), 'The gut–brain axis: interactions between enteric microbiota, central and enteric nervous systems': www.ncbi.nlm.nih.gov/pubmed/25830558

96. Ma, Q., et al. (2019), 'Impact of microbiota on central nervous system and neurological diseases: the gut–brain axis': https://jneuroinflammation.biomedcentral.com/articles/10.1186/s12974-019-1434-3

97. Bischoff, S.C., et al. (2014), 'Intestinal permeability – a new target for disease prevention and therapy': www.ncbi.nlm.nih.gov/pmc/articles/PMC4253991/

98. Li, Y, et al. (2018), 'The Role of Microbiome in Insomnia, Circadian Disturbance and Depression', *Frontiers in Psychiatry*, 9(December):1–11.

99. Appleton, J. (2018), 'The Gut–Brain Axis: Influence of Microbiota on Mood and Mental Health': www.ncbi.nlm.nih.gov/pmc/articles/PMC6469458/

100. D'Mello, C., et al. (2015), 'Probiotics Improve Inflammation-Associated Sickness Behavior by Altering Communication between

the Peripheral Immune System and the Brain': www.jneurosci.org/content/35/30/10821.full

101. Ganci, M., et al. (2019), 'The role of the brain–gut–microbiota axis in psychology: The importance of considering gut microbiota in the development, perpetuation, and treatment of psychological disorders': www.ncbi.nlm.nih.gov/pmc/articles/PMC6851798/

102. Parkar, S.G., et al. (2019), 'Potential role for the gut microbiota in modulating host circadian rhythms and metabolic health', *Microorganisms*, 7(2):1–21.

103. Fasano, A. (2020), 'All disease begins in the (leaky) gut: role of zonulin-mediated gut permeability in the pathogenesis of some chronic inflammatory diseases': www.ncbi.nlm.nih.gov/pubmed/32051759F1000

104. Kolacz, J. and Porges, S.W. (2018), 'Chronic Diffuse Pain and Functional Gastrointestinal Disorders After Traumatic Stress: Pathophysiology Through a Polyvagal Perspective': www.ncbi.nlm.nih.gov/pubmed/29904631

105. Maes, M. and Twisk, F.N. (2009), 'Why myalgic encephalomyelitis/chronic fatigue syndrome (ME/CFS) may kill you: disorders in the inflammatory and oxidative and nitrosative stress (IO&NS) pathways may explain cardiovascular disorders in ME/CFS': www.ncbi.nlm.nih.gov/pubmed/20038921

106. Maes, M. (2009), 'Inflammatory and oxidative and nitrosative stress pathways underpinning chronic fatigue, somatization and psychosomatic symptoms': www.ncbi.nlm.nih.gov/pubmed/19127706

107. Yu, LC-H. (2018), 'Microbiota dysbiosis and barrier dysfunction in inflammatory bowel disease and colorectal cancers: exploring a common ground hypothesis': www.ncbi.nlm.nih.gov/pmc/articles/PMC6234774/

108. Bures, J., et al. (2006), 'Small intestinal bacterial overgrowth syndrome', *World Journal of Gastroenterology*, 16(24):2978–90.

109. Saffouri, G.B., et al. (2019), 'Small intestinal microbial dysbiosis underlies symptoms associated with functional gastrointestinal disorders': www.ncbi.nlm.nih.gov/pmc/articles/PMC6494866/

110. Sachdev, A.H. and Pimentel, M. (2013), 'Gastrointestinal bacterial overgrowth: pathogenesis and clinical significance': www.ncbi.nlm.nih.gov/pubmed/23997926

111. Pimentel, M., et al. (2004), 'A link between irritable bowel syndrome and fibromyalgia may be related to findings on lactulose breath testing': www.ncbi.nlm.nih.gov/pubmed/15020342

Chapter 10: Your Hormones and Your Body's Energy Reserve System

112. Cadegiani, F.A. and Kater, C.E. (2016), 'Adrenal fatigue does not exist: a systematic review': www.ncbi.nlm.nih.gov/pmc/articles/PMC4997656/

113. Wyller, V.B., et al. (2016), 'Altered neuroendocrine control and association to clinical symptoms in adolescent chronic fatigue syndrome: a cross-sectional study': www.ncbi.nlm.nih.gov/pubmed/27149955

114. Torres-Harding, S., et al. (2008), 'The associations between basal salivary cortisol and illness symptomatology in chronic fatigue syndrome': www.ncbi.nlm.nih.gov/pmc/articles/PMC2730359/

115. Ludwig, D.S. (2014), 'Clinical update: the low-glycaemic-index diet. https://www.thelancet.com/journals/lancet/article/PIIS0140-6736%2807%2960427-9/fulltext

116. Savage, D.B., et al. (2007), 'Disordered Lipid Metabolism and the Pathogenesis of Insulin Resistance': www.ncbi.nlm.nih.gov/pmc/articles/PMC2995548/

117. Moghaddam, E., et al. (2006), 'The Effects of Fat and Protein on Glycemic Responses in Nondiabetic Humans Vary with Waist Circumference, Fasting Plasma Insulin, and Dietary Fiber Intake': https://academic.oup.com/jn/article/136/10/2506/4746688

118. Hucklebridge, F., et al. (2005), 'The diurnal patterns of the adrenal steroids cortisol and dehydroepiandrosterone (DHEA) in relation to awakening': www.sciencedirect.com/science/article/abs/pii/S030645300400071X

119. Arendt, J. (2006), 'Melatonin and Human Rhythms': www.tandfonline.com/doi/full/10.1080/07420520500464361

120. Pevet, P. and Challet, E. (2011), 'Melatonin: Both master clock output and internal time-giver in the circadian clocks network':

www.sciencedirect.com/science/article/abs/pii/S09284257
11000040?via%3Dihub

121. Videnovic, A., et al. (2014), 'Circadian melatonin rhythm and excessive daytime sleepiness in Parkinson disease': www.ncbi.nlm.nih.gov/pubmed/24566763JAMA

122. Tsang, A., et al. (2014), 'Interactions between endocrine and circadian systems': https://jme.bioscientifica.com/view/journals/jme/52/1/R1.xml

123. Cajochen, C., et al. (2011), 'Evening exposure to a light-emitting diodes (LED)-backlit computer screen affects circadian physiology and cognitive performance': www.physiology.org/doi/10.1152/japplphysiol.00165.2011

124. 124 Cajochen, C., et al. (2005) 'High Sensitivity of Human Melatonin, Alertness, Thermoregulation, and Heart Rate to Short Wavelength Light': https://pubmed.ncbi.nlm.nih.gov/15585546/2005

125. Schmidt, C., et al. (2018), 'Light exposure via a head-mounted device suppresses melatonin and improves vigilant attention without affecting cortisol and comfort': https://orbi.uliege.be/bitstream/2268/226193/1/Schmidt 2018 PsyCh.pdf

126. Green, A., et al. (2017), 'Evening light exposure to computer screens disrupts human sleep, biological rhythms, and attention abilities': www.tandfonline.com/doi/full/10.1080/07420528.2017.1324878

127. Cho, Y, et al. (2016), 'Effects of artificial light at night on human health: A literature review of observational and experimental studies applied to exposure assessment': www.ncbi.nlm.nih.gov/pubmed/26375320

128. Codoñer-Franch, P. and Gombert, M. (2018), 'Circadian rhythms in the pathogenesis of gastrointestinal diseases', *World Journal of Gastroenterology*, 24(38):4297–4303.

129. Tähkämö, L., et al. (2019), 'Systematic review of light exposure impact on human circadian rhythm': www.tandfonline.com/doi/full/10.1080/07420528.2018.1527773

130. Prayag, A., et al. (2019), 'Light Modulation of Human Clocks, Wake, and Sleep': www.mdpi.com/2624-5175/1/1/17

131. Leese, G., et al. (1996), 'Short-term night-shift working mimics the pituitary-adrenocortical dysfunction in chronic fatigue syndrome':

https://academic.oup.com/jcem/article-lookup/doi/10.1210/
jcem.81.5.8626849

Chapter 11: Your Immune System – Reducing Your Body's Load

132. Cressey, D. (2011), 'XMRV paper withdrawn': http://blogs.nature.com/
news/2011/12/xmrv-paper-withdrawn.html

133. Anand, S.K. and Tikoo, S.K. (2013), 'Viruses as Modulators of
Mitochondrial Functions', *Advances in Virology*, vol. 2013, Article ID
738794

134. Centers for Disease Control and Prevention (2018), 'Possible Causes |
Myalgic Encephalomyelitis/Chronic Fatigue Syndrome (ME/CFS)':
www.cdc.gov/me-cfs/about/possible-causes.html

135. Ikuta, K., et al. (2003), 'Diagnostic evaluation of 2', 5'-oligoadenylate
synthetase activities and antibodies against Epstein-Barr virus
and *Coxiella burnetii* in patients with chronic fatigue syndrome
in Japan': www.sciencedirect.com/science/article/abs/pii/
S1286457903002193?via%3Dihub

136. Eriksen, W. (2018), 'ME/CFS, case definition, and serological response
to Epstein-Barr virus. A systematic literature review': www.tandfonline.
com/doi/full/10.1080/21641846.2018.1503125

137. Rasa, S., et al. (2018), 'Chronic viral infections in myalgic
encephalomyelitis/chronic fatigue syndrome (ME/CFS)': https://www.
ncbi.nlm.nih.gov/pmc/articles/PMC6167797/

138. Yalcin, S., et al. (1994), 'Prevalence of Human Herpesvirus 6 Variants
A and B in Patients with Chronic Fatigue Syndrome': http://doi.wiley.
com/10.1111/j.1348-0421.1994.tb01827.x

139. Eldin, C., et al. (2017), 'From Q Fever to Coxiella burnetii Infection: a
Paradigm Change': www.ncbi.nlm.nih.gov/pubmed/27856520 2017

140. Buchwald, D., et al. (1996), 'Viral serologies in patients with
chronic fatigue and chronic fatigue syndrome': http://doi.wiley.
com/10.1002/%28SICI%291096-9071%28199609%2950%3A1%3C2
5%3A%3AAID-JMV6%3E3.0.CO%3B2-V

141. Koelle, D.M., et al (2002), 'Markers of Viral Infection in Monozygotic Twins Discordant for Chronic Fatigue Syndrome': https://academic.oup.com/cid/article-lookup/doi/10.1086/341774

142. Brewer, J.H., et al. (2013), 'Detection of Mycotoxins in Patients with Chronic Fatigue Syndrome': www.ncbi.nlm.nih.gov/pmc/articles/PMC3705282/

143. Chester, A.C. and Levine, P.H. (1994), 'Concurrent Sick Building Syndrome and Chronic Fatigue Syndrome: Epidemic Neuromyasthenia Revisited': http://academic.oup.com/cid/article/18/Supplement_1/S43/317008/Concurrent-Sick-Building-Syndrome-and-Chronic

144. Campbell, A.W., et al. (2004), 'Mold and Mycotoxins: Effects on the Neurological and Immune Systems in Humans': www.sciencedirect.com/science/article/pii/S0065216404550153?via%3Dihub Adv

145. Rea, W.J., et al. (2003), 'Effects of Toxic Exposure to Molds and Mycotoxins in Building-Related Illnesses': https://pubmed.ncbi.nlm.nih.gov/15143852/

146. Ratnaseelan, A.M, et al. (2018), 'Effects of Mycotoxins on Neuropsychiatric Symptoms and Immune Processes': www.clinicaltherapeutics.com/article/S0149-2918(18)30229-7/fulltext

147. Centers for Disease Control and Prevention (2019), 'Lyme and Other Tickborne Diseases Increasing': www.cdc.gov/media/dpk/diseases-and-conditions/lyme-disease/index.html

Chapter 13: Learning to Listen to Your Body

148. White, P.D., et al. (2011), 'Comparison of adaptive pacing therapy, cognitive behaviour therapy, graded exercise therapy, and specialist medical care for chronic fatigue syndrome (PACE): a randomised trial': www.ncbi.nlm.nih.gov/pubmed/21334061

149. Wilshire, C., et al. (2017), 'Can patients with chronic fatigue syndrome really recover after graded exercise or cognitive behavioural therapy? A critical commentary and preliminary re-analysis of the PACE trial': www.tandfonline.com/doi/full/10.1080/21641846.2017.1259724

150. Wilshire, C.E., et al. (2018), 'Rethinking the treatment of chronic fatigue syndrome – a reanalysis and evaluation of findings from a

recent major trial of graded exercise and CBT': www.ncbi.nlm.nih.gov/pubmed/29562932BMC

151. Sharpe, M., et al. (2019), 'The PACE trial of treatments for chronic fatigue syndrome: a response to Wilshire et al.': www.ncbi.nlm.nih.gov/pubmed/30871632

152. Wilshire, C.E. and Kindlon, T. (2019), 'Response: Sharpe, Goldsmith and Chalder fail to restore confidence in the PACE trial findings': www.ncbi.nlm.nih.gov/pubmed/30914065

153. Torjesen, I. (2015), 'Tackling fears about exercise is important for ME treatment, analysis indicates': www.bmj.com/cgi/doi/10.1136/bmj.h227

154. Twisk, F. and Maes, M. (2009), 'A review on cognitive behavorial therapy (CBT) and graded exercise therapy (GET) in myalgic encephalomyelitis (ME)/chronic fatigue syndrome (CFS): CBT/GET is not only ineffective and not evidence-based, but also potentially harmful for many patients with ME/CFS': www.researchgate.net/publication/38034776_A_review_on_cognitive_behavorial_therapy_CBT_and_graded_exercise_therapy_GET_in_myalgic_encephalomyelitis_ME_chronic_fatigue_syndrome_CFS_CBTGET_is_not_only_ineffective_and_not_evidence-based_but_also

Chapter 15: Cultivating a Healing State

155. Lardone, A. et al. (2018), 'Mindfulness Meditation Is Related to Long-Lasting Changes in Hippocampal Functional Topology during Resting State: A Magnetoencephalography Study': www.ncbi.nlm.nih.gov/pmc/articles/PMC6312586/

156. Braboszcz, C., et al. (2017), 'Increased Gamma Brainwave Amplitude Compared to Control in Three Different Meditation Traditions': www.ncbi.nlm.nih.gov/pmc/articles/PMC5261734/

157. Cahn, B.R., et al. (2013), 'Event-related delta, theta, alpha and gamma correlates to auditory oddball processing during Vipassana meditation': www.ncbi.nlm.nih.gov/pmc/articles/PMC3541491/

158. Amihai, I. and Kozhevnikov, M. (2014), 'Arousal vs. Relaxation: A Comparison of the Neurophysiological and Cognitive Correlates of Vajrayana and Theravada Meditative Practices': www.ncbi.nlm.nih.gov/pmc/articles/PMC4106862/

159. Fucci, E., et al. (2018), 'Differential effects of non-dual and focused attention meditations on the formation of automatic perceptual habits in expert practitioners': www.ncbi.nlm.nih.gov/pmc/articles/PMC7050275/

Chapter 16: Nutrition Fundamentals

160. Guandalini, S. and Newland C. (2011), 'Differentiating Food Allergies from Food Intolerances': http://link.springer.com/10.1007/s11894-011-0215-7

161. Tuck, C.J., et al. (2019), 'Food Intolerances': www.ncbi.nlm.nih.gov/pmc/articles/PMC6682924/

162. Lomer, M.C.E. (2015), 'Review article: the aetiology, diagnosis, mechanisms and clinical evidence for food intolerance': http://doi.wiley.com/10.1111/apt.13041

163. Layman, D.K., et al. (2003), 'A Reduced Ratio of Dietary Carbohydrate to Protein Improves Body Composition and Blood Lipid Profiles during Weight Loss in Adult Women': https://academic.oup.com/jn/article/133/2/411/4687883

164. Puri, B.K. (2007), 'Long-chain polyunsaturated fatty acids and the pathophysiology of myalgic encephalomyelitis (chronic fatigue syndrome), *Journal Clinical Pathology*, 60(2):122–4.

165. BANT (British Assocation for Applied Nutrition and Nutritional Therapy) (2015), 'EAT A RAINBOW – 7 A DAY': https://bant.org.uk/wp-content/uploads/2015/09/EAT_A_RAINBOW_GUIDELINES.pdf

166. Venturini, L., et al. (2019), 'Modification of Immunological Parameters, Oxidative Stress Markers, Mood Symptoms, and Well-Being Status in CFS Patients after Probiotic Intake: Observations from a Pilot Study': www.ncbi.nlm.nih.gov/pmc/articles/PMC6906814/

167. Galland, L. (2014), 'The Gut Microbiome and the Brain': www.ncbi.nlm.nih.gov/pmc/articles/PMC4259177/

168. Lakhan, S.E. and Kirchgessner A. (2010), 'Gut inflammation in chronic fatigue syndrome': https://pubmed.ncbi.nlm.nih.gov/20939923/

169. Holmstrup, M.E, et al. (2010), 'Effect of meal frequency on glucose and insulin excursions over the course of a day': www.sciencedirect.com/science/article/abs/pii/S1751499110000545

170. Mattson, M.P., et al. (2017), 'Impact of intermittent fasting on health and disease processes': www.ncbi.nlm.nih.gov/pmc/articles/PMC5411330/

171. Anton, S.D., et al. (2018), 'Flipping the Metabolic Switch: Understanding and Applying Health Benefits of Fasting': www.ncbi.nlm.nih.gov/pmc/articles/PMC5783752/

172. Crinnion, W. (2015), 'Organic Foods Contain Higher Levels of Certain Nutrients, Lower Levels of Pesticides, and May Provide Health Benefits for the Consumer': http://archive.foundationalmedicinereview.com/publications/15/1/4.pdf

173. Benelam, B. and Wyness L. (2010), 'Hydration and health: a review': http://doi.wiley.com/10.1111/j.1467-3010.2009.01795.x

174. Miquel-Kergoat, S., et al. (2015), 'Effects of chewing on appetite, food intake and gut hormones: A systematic review and meta-analysis': www.sciencedirect.com/science/article/pii/S0031938415300317?via%3Dihub

175. Giacco, R., et al. (2014), 'A whole-grain cereal-based diet lowers postprandial plasma insulin and triglyceride levels in individuals with metabolic syndrome': www.sciencedirect.com/science/article/abs/pii/S0939475314000386

176. Catassi, C., et al. (2013), 'Non-Celiac Gluten Sensitivity: The New Frontier of Gluten Related Disorders': www.mdpi.com/2072-6643/5/10/3839/htm

177. Elli, L., et al. (2016), 'Evidence for the Presence of Non-Celiac Gluten Sensitivity in Patients with Functional Gastrointestinal Symptoms: Results from a Multicenter Randomized Double-Blind Placebo-Controlled Gluten Challenge': www.ncbi.nlm.nih.gov/pubmed/26867199

178. Vojdani, A., et al. (2014), 'The Prevalence of Antibodies against Wheat and Milk Proteins in Blood Donors and Their Contribution to Neuroimmune Reactivities': www.ncbi.nlm.nih.gov/pmc/articles/PMC3916846/

179. Misselwitz, B., et al. (2019), 'Update on lactose malabsorption and intolerance: pathogenesis, diagnosis and clinical management': http://gut.bmj.com/lookup/doi/10.1136/gutjnl-2019-318404

180. Corti, R., et al. (2002), 'Coffee Acutely Increases Sympathetic Nerve Activity and Blood Pressure Independently of Caffeine Content': www.ahajournals.org/doi/10.1161/01.CIR.0000046228.97025.3A

181. Bunsawat, K., (2015), 'Caffeine delays autonomic recovery following acute exercise': http://journals.sagepub.com/doi/10.1177/2047487314554867

182. Ramalakshmi, K. and Raghavan, B. (1999), 'Caffeine in Coffee: Its Removal. Why and How?' www.tandfonline.com/doi/abs/10.1080/10408699991279231

183. Lovallo, W.R. et al. (2005), 'Caffeine Stimulation of Cortisol Secretion Across the Waking Hours in Relation to Caffeine Intake Levels': www.ncbi.nlm.nih.gov/pmc/articles/PMC2257922/

▪▪ ACKNOWLEDGMENTS ▪▪

If I was to thank everyone who has played a role in shaping the theories and insights shared in this book, I think you would give up reading before we even reached the first chapter. So, I'll keep this is as brief as I can.

From the thousands of patients we have had the privilege to support over the years, to the incredible practitioners past and present who make up the Optimum Health Clinic (OHC) teams, each of you has played a role in evolving, confirming, and challenging the wisdom shared in this book. Thank you.

Although the words you read in these pages are my own, this book was a team effort in every way, from the years of development of the ideas at The Optimum Health Clinic, to the synthesizing of these ideas into this book you are reading.

I particularly want to thank Niki Gratrix and Anna Duschinsky who co-founded OHC with me back in 2004. It was a crazy time, and we had a lot to learn along the way. But our core values of an integrative approach with the patient at the heart of it has only become more deeply confirmed in its wisdom as the years have passed.

Our various department directors – former and current – Jess Thompson, Sara Jackson, Bebe Kohlap, Tanya Page, and Helen Lynam, thank you for your enormous efforts and lasting friendship. Particularly, I want to thank our CEO Kirsty Cullen for her dedication to the mission of OHC, and loyalty to our core values and purpose.

I must also acknowledge my PA Grace Allen, and our finance/operations manager Glynn Gratrix. Your patience and steadfastness in keeping the potential chaos of my business life on track is hugely appreciated and what allowed me the time to write this book. Thank you also to the trustees of our registered charity David Butcher and Ian Hatton, I greatly appreciate your support and efforts over the years.

I always say it is the people that make OHC the place it is, thank you all for playing your part in that.

Thank you to my commissioning editors Elaine O'Neill and Emily Arbis for believing in this book and guiding me along the way, and huge thanks to my editor, Debra Wolter, for her consistently helpful suggestions, and managing editor, Julie Oughton, for supervising the book to fruition. Thank you to the various Hay House teams for being such as a delight to work with. My deep thanks also to Kelly Notaras for being a champion of my writing long before this book came to life, and Michelle Pilley for having faith in me.

On my internal editing team, thank you particularly to Sarah Benjamins for her many hours of research to confirm, support, and challenge my ideas, and to Kirsty Cullen, Claire Sehinson, and Helen Lynam for enthusiastically and patiently feeding back on my drafts along the way.

Finally, and most importantly, I want to thank my ever supportive and loving wife, Tania, along with our three beautiful girls, Marli, Ariella, and Lyra. Your love and support is what makes all that I do possible.

·· INDEX ··

articles 11, 127, 154
see also individual publications
'As if' frame 88–9
athletes
  levels of ATP in 31
autoimmune disease 25

B
Babesiosis 135
bacteria 133, 134
  gut 103, 106, 109–10, 111, 121, 195, 198
Bartonellosis 135
belief, the power of 142–3, 148–50
biomarkers for disease 20, 25
blood sugar 120–21, 188, 190–91
  impact on energy levels 120
  balancing 121, 193–4
  rollercoaster 191–2
blood tests 25, 220
  full blood count 25
  kidney function 25
  liver function 25
  Lyme disease 134
  mitochondrial function 38, 46
  thyroid 25
bodily systems 51, 54–5
  digestive system 33, 93, 101–104, 104–108, 122
  endocrine system 55, 116–25 *see also* hormones
  immune system 44, 103, 108, 127–37, 192, 214
  nervous system 46–8, 68–70, 88–99, 103, 106, 166–7, 178–82
bowel movements 110, 111, 113
brain fog 103, 104, 113, 132, 159, 192, 193
British Medical Journal Open 11

C
caffeine 94, 115–17, 119, 197
campaigning 21
'canary in the coal mine' analogy 47
cancer 25, 78, 83
  stomach 107, 112
candida 109, 111
carbohydrates 33, 120, 121, 189–92
  refined 110, 119, 189–91, 196
  unrefined 196
caregivers 45
  advice for 12–13
case studies
  Alex 3–9, 17–18, 71–2, 142–4, 187–9
  Anna 66
  Claire 61–4, 66, 70, 75–6
  Colin 87–90, 96, 175
  David 77–9, 86
  James 163, 173
  Karen 115–17
  Louise 45–6
  Monica 146
  Nick 41–3, 55
  Niki 188–9
  Violet 218–21
celiac disease 25
cell danger response theory (CDR) 46–8
Centers for Disease Control and Prevention (CDC) 21, 80
childhood
  development of personality patterns 72, 82
  trauma 79–80, 82, 96 *see also* adverse childhood experiences (ACEs)
chronic fatigue syndrome (CFS) 4, 10, 13, 64
  acceptance by medical community 21, 150

energy depleting psychologies 53,
64–8
see also personality patterns
energy drinks 115, 119, 197
Epstein-Barr *see* glandular fever
exercise 31, 36, 44
as a stimulant 117
fatigue after 30, 35–6 *see also*
post-exertional malaise
timing of 122

F
fasting, intermittent 195
fatigue
4 types of 159–61
adrenal 118, 122, 188
'all in the mind' 20–21, 43–4,
150, 153, 156
as a symptom 24
attitude of others to 17, 83, 153
causes of 37, 51–5, 117, 129–30
definition 24
emotional effects of 5–6, 82–3,
163
holistic approach to 23, 128
mild 13, 115, 173
misdiagnosis as depression 44, 153
recovery from 9, 39, 73, 122,
141–50, 164–74, 211–16
relapse 63–4, 72, 150
research into 21, 38, 51, 127–9,
130, 154–5
role of genetics in 51–2
role of personality in 53, 63–76
specific illnesses 13
symptoms of 25, 44, 78, 159
see also fatigue-related conditions;
fatigue symptoms
fatigue mapping 50–58
fatigue map 1 52–5
fatigue map 2 56–8, 141

fatigue-related conditions 13
acceptance by medical community
21
biomarkers for 20, 25
conventional treatments for
154–6
diagnosis 24–7
diagnostic process 25–6
fatigue sufferers
campaigning by 21–2
disability payments for 156
experience of 15, 22
fatigue symptoms
brain fog 103, 104, 113, 132, 159,
192, 193
depression 43–4
digestive symptoms 101, 108
disordered sleep 25, 165
dizziness 4, 25, 134
'leaky gut' 108
muscle pain 25
fats 194
sources of 194
Felitti, Vincent 80
fiber 112, 121, 190, 195
sources of 197
fight, flight or freeze response 91–3,
106
Fitzgerald, Dr. Kara 52
fluid intake 112, 196
FODMAP diet 110
food
as source of energy 33, 191
organic 195
processed 198
to avoid 196–8
see also diet
food intolerances 107–108, 121,
192–3
symptoms of 192, 193
functional medicine
definition 23

R
radical responsibility 13, 14, 147, 212
Ramsay, Dr. Melvin 19
recovery 9, 39, 56–8, 73, 141–50
  3Ds to success 142–50
  goals 215–17
  plan for 56–8, 211–16
  relapse in 63–4, 72–3, 150, 166
  sequencing of 57–8
  stages of 57, 164–74
relapse 63–4, 72–3, 150, 166
research
  flaws in 127–9, 130, 154–6
  personal 207
  published studies 11, 127,
   154–6
RESET program 98
Ross River virus 130
Royal Free Disease
  outbreak 18–19
  psychiatric diagnosis 21
  research into 21
Royal Free Hospital, London 18–19
  see also Royal Free Disease
rubella 130

S
Schneider, Meir 143–4
Science 127
screens 123–4
Selye, Hans 90
Shoemaker, Dr. Ritchie 131
sleep
  brainwaves during 177–8
  circadian rhythms 122–4
  for healing 165, 177–8
  hygiene 126, 131
  poor 25, 39, 80, 98, 135, 166
  role of hormones in 122–3, 124
  see also sleep disorders; insomnia
sleep disorders 25, 80

small intestinal bacterial overgrowth
  (SIBO) 109, 113, 121
small intestine 107–110
social media 94, 206
specialist medical care (SMC) 154
Stachybotrys atra 131
Stachybotrys chartarum 131
stimulants 115–16, 117, 197
  reducing 119, 197
stomach 106–107, 112–13
  cancer 107, 112
  conditions 107
stress
  3 types of 90–91
  biological origin of 91–3
  caused by fatigue 95, 169
  definition 90
  impact on energy production 45–7
  impact on healing 44–5
  impact on hormones 119
  impact on immune system 44
  modern sources of 94–5
  normalizing 94–5
  response to 91–3, 97, 116
  see also maladaptive stress response
   (MSR); 'loads'; stress state;
   trauma
stress state 93–4, 97–9, 169, 177–8,
  181
sugar 110, 115, 119, 196
  see also blood sugar
sunlight 123
supplements 39, 125, 131, 144
  co-enzyme Q-10 39
  colostrum 131
  D-ribose 39
  L-carnitine 39
  magnesium 39, 125
  pantothenic acid 125
  Vitamin C 125, 131
  Vitamin D 131
  zinc 131

ABOUT THE AUTHOR

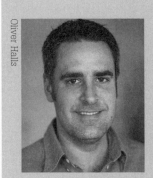

Oliver Halls

Alex Howard is the Founder and Chairman of The Optimum Health Clinic (OHC), one of the world's leading integrative medicine clinics specializing in fatigue. With a team of 20 full-time practitioners supporting thousands of patients in 50+ countries, the OHC team have pioneered working with patients remotely since 2005.

Along with founding and leading the OHC practitioner teams for the past 17 years, Alex is an immensely experienced psychology practitioner, having delivered over 10,000 consultations. He has also led the Therapeutic Coaching practitioner programme since 2005, training the next generation of psychology practitioners. Since March 2020, Alex has been documenting his therapeutic work with real-life patients via his *In Therapy with Alex Howard* YouTube series.

In 2015, Alex founded the leading online video platform Conscious Life, which has produced programs with over 150 teachers, including Byron Katie, Marianne Williamson, Dr. Joe Dispenza, and Ken Wilber. In the last few years, Alex has created some of the largest online conferences in the health and mind–body markets, including the Fatigue Super Conference and the Trauma and Mind–Body Super Conference. Alex's online conferences have been attended by over a quarter of a million people.

Alex is also the author of *Why Me?: My Journey from ME to Health and Happiness.*

 alexhowardtv

 @alexhowardtherapy

 alexhowardtv

www.alexhoward.com

255

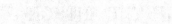

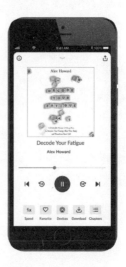

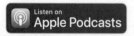

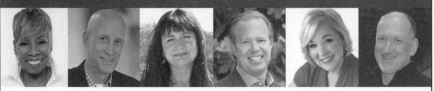

HAY HOUSE
Look within

Join the conversation about latest products,
events, exclusive offers and more.

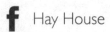 Hay House

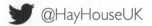 @HayHouseUK

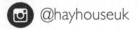 @hayhouseuk

We'd love to hear from you!